# 30-Something and the Clock is Ticking

# 30 Something and the Clock is Ticking

## What Happens When You Can No Longer Ignore the Baby Issue

## KASEY EDWARDS

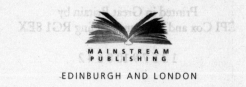

**MAINSTREAM PUBLISHING**

EDINBURGH AND LONDON

First published in Great Britain in 2011 by
MAINSTREAM PUBLISHING COMPANY
(EDINBURGH) LTD
7 Albany Street
Edinburgh EH1 3UG

ISBN 9781845967345

This book is substantially a work of non-fiction based on the life
experiences and recollections of the author. In some limited cases,
names and descriptions of people, places and the detail of events
have been changed for artistic purposes and to protect
the privacy of others.

A catalogue record for this book is available
from the British Library

To my lovely Christopher. Without your boundless love, humour and support, this story, and the telling of it, would not have been possible.

# CONTENTS

# INTRODUCTION

## Facing the baby question

Have you ever seriously thought about whether or not you want to have a baby? Have you wondered what it would mean to you? To your career, your body, your relationships, your mental health? I'm not talking about when your period was late after that tipsy evening when you ended up in bed with Mr Oh-So-Right-But-Only-For-One-Night, or about those neurotic moments when you contemplated sticking holes in the condom when the love of your life (or so he seemed at the time) wouldn't marry you. I'm not even referring to the fantasy of getting knocked up so you could legitimately quit your job and opt out of the workforce for a while. I'm talking about that moment when your fertility train is chugging out of the station and you've got one foot aboard and one foot firmly, stubbornly planted on the platform.

I have.

For a long time, my views on babies were firmly set. In my teens and 20s, I was anti-kids. I was one of those feminists who arrogantly believed I was meant for far greater things than 'just' being a breeder. I couldn't reconcile the inequality of motherhood. Why should the woman have to carry the child for nine months? Why should she have to endure childbirth, get saggy boobs from breastfeeding and sacrifice her career, identity and pelvic-floor muscles when all the man has to do is cum? I didn't consider motherhood as any sort of accomplishment, because, after all, anybody could do it. It was the great leveller of all women. It didn't matter how hard you studied, how hard you worked or what the title was on your business card. Anyone who could get a man to sleep with them could have a baby. And, let's face it, that's hardly an achievement.

As my 30s approached, I started to soften my stance. Other people's babies started to look quite cute – so long as I didn't have to touch them. I used to hate it when people would thrust their baby into my lap. I'd sit there tensely, trying not to break it, wondering how long social etiquette dictated I should hold it before giving it back without causing offence. All the time I was secretly thinking that they should hold their own bloody baby. It frustrated me that babies were so useless. I mean, babies can't do anything for themselves, and until they understand object permanence and the relationship between cause and effect, it's impossible to relate to them. And then, the certainty that I never wanted a baby, which had been a landmark of my youth, began to erode – if ever so slightly.

I figured this was no big deal. I was only 32 years old, which left plenty of time to make up my mind about the baby question. I decided I didn't need to think about it until the day when the urge to have a baby was greater than the urge not to. And if that urge never came, then so be it. I would be happily childless and embrace my independence, my disposable income and a belly without stretch marks.

Imagine my surprise when one day I was talking to my boyfriend Chris and the words 'I want to have a baby' vomited out of my mouth. It was almost like the words were sent directly from my ovaries to my mouth and had bypassed my brain. (I'll be sure to be less judgemental next time I accuse a man of thinking with his dick.) What was I thinking? I'd only known Chris for a year. Sure, we were serious and had recently started living together, but that conversation was still far off in some distant future. And the timing was terrible. Our apartment was a shoebox, far too small to fit a baby and all the brightly coloured plastic stuff babies seem to attract. Our savings were even tinier. I quickly retracted the statement and agreed with Chris that we would discuss the baby subject again in a year, and not a moment sooner.

Less than two weeks later, after a visit to my gynaecologist, we could talk of nothing else. My fertility train had started its engine and the conductor had shouted, 'All aboard!' I was too young to deal with this. Crunch time had come, by my estimation, about ten years ahead of schedule.

In the months that followed, I was forced to contemplate all those baby questions that used to bore me to tears if I was trapped at the clucky end of the table at a dinner party. What would it mean to want a baby but be unable to have one? Would it leave a void that I could never fill with a couple of fluffy white mutts and designer handbags? Would my life be ruined? Or what would it be like if I did have a baby only to discover that I didn't want it, that I preferred my life before? I'd be stuck with a baby for ever, unable to give it back. Would my life be ruined?

Faced with the biggest decision of my life, I decided to do some research and some soul-searching to help me decide. I wanted to uncover the truth about motherhood, without the sugar coating. I wanted to know about all the things people don't talk about because it's socially awkward to do so or they'd just prefer to forget. I wanted to know definitively, and ahead of time, if my life would be better or worse if I had a child. What would I be giving up, what would I be gaining and what would I regret? I spoke to people who had children and to people who didn't, people who were infertile and never had the luxury of choosing, and people who had all the right plumbing but no ready access to sperm. Along the way I discovered how the desire for a baby can drive people to the brink of insanity, and perhaps over the edge; the logistical challenges presented when ovulating and trying to conceive on a long-haul flight (for the first time I appreciated what a huge achievement membership of the mile high club really is, given the size of aeroplane toilets); the indignity and despair of IVF; and the price of buying sperm on the Internet.

Most of all, I found that at some point in every woman's life we all have to face the baby question. For some, it's fleeting and the answer is obvious. For other women, the question creeps up slowly and the answer is heart-wrenchingly painful. There is no single right answer, but what I did discover is that, regardless of the answer, it's a lot better to face the question head-on and on our own terms rather than let time, ignorance and social pressures make the decision for us. This is my story and the stories of other women about what we decided, what we were unable to decide and how we dealt with the consequences.

# 1

# TICK TOCK YOUR EGGS ARE POX

She is coming towards me holding something that looks a lot like a vibrator, and the business end is pointed at me. But it isn't a vibrator. For a start, where are the bunny ears and the multiple-speed setting, not to mention the glitter encased within pink silicone gel? (Every vibrator should be covered in glitter in my opinion.) Not only is this device not covered in glitter, it doesn't look nearly as much fun.

No, this isn't an episode of lesbian experimentation. It is a visit to my gynaecologist. There are few things in my life that I hate more than having a smear test. Surely there has to be an easier way than having a cold metallic duck bill smothered in KY stuck inside you. And it's the only time in my life when I put up with being naked in a room with fluorescent lighting. Every year I am horrified by my dimply skin under the bright lights and resolve never to eat chocolate again.

I'm about to swing off the bed and reach for my underwear when my gynaecologist Dr Lucy holds up her evil twin of the vibrator and issues those ten fateful words that will change my life. 'While you're here,' she says, casual as you like, 'I may as well check your ovaries.'

I'm about to decline. Why does she need to check my ovaries? I've got them – two of them, in fact, just as the owner's manual says I should. I know this because without fail I get a twingey pain in them every month when I ovulate. And I feel certain that checking my ovaries is going to involve having something else shoved up me. Sensing my reluctance, Dr Lucy stands between me and my knickers. 'This won't hurt,' she lies.

Dr Lucy has been my gynaecologist for years. She's also one of the few female doctors to specialise in fertility. When the crusty old male gatekeepers of her profession refused to allow her to train under them, she wasn't deterred. She relocated her family to the US for a few years so she could do her training there. I like her because she dared to break the mould of her profession. She's fun, funky, feminine and doesn't take shit from anyone. She also has a wardrobe to die for.

I reluctantly lie back on the bed and try to focus on Dr Lucy's six-inch heels rather than the vibrator doppelgänger she's using for my internal ovary scan. Surely her feet must be killing her at the end of each day. Dr Lucy starts counting. 'One, two, three, four . . .' She stops when she gets to twenty.

'Twenty what?' I ask.

'You have twenty follicles on your right ovary,' she says.

'How many am I supposed to have?'

'About ten.'

For a moment, I'm well pleased with myself. I love being an overachiever. Twenty has got to be better than ten, right? Then Dr Lucy explains the principle of quality over quantity. Every month your ovaries alternate in producing eggs. Each follicle in the ovary produces an egg and then, a few days before you ovulate, your body selects the best egg in the ovary to continue growing and ditches the rest. Rather than producing approximately ten decent eggs, my right ovary is producing twenty crappy, poor-quality eggs. My body is spreading its resources so thinly that when it selects the best egg out of the twenty, it's still not very good. Most likely the quality will be too poor to make a baby.

'Lucky I have another ovary then,' I say hopefully.

My optimism is short-lived. Dr Lucy scans my left ovary and finds the correct number of follicles. Yay for the left ovary! And then Dr Lucy tells me about the cyst. 'It could be nothing,' she says. 'But it might be something, so I'd better go in and take a look. I can operate on you next week.'

'Could it be cancer?' I ask.

'Unlikely.'

'Well, I've got nothing to worry about then,' I say in blissful ignorance.

As soon as I leave Dr Lucy's room, and having arranged to go in for surgery, I phone my best friend Emma. Emma and I went to the same high school. She was a year above me, but I met her when we were both cast in the school musical, *Bad Boys*. Emma had a lead role as Tallulah, a sexy little tramp with a feather boa, and I played a dumb gangster who said two lines and was then killed with a cream pie. I like to think that Garbo would have died to say those two lines as well as I did and that my Shakespearean death, which took longer than delivering the lines, was worthy of The Globe.

When I say I got to know Emma during the musical, what I actually mean is that I got to know of her during the musical. She was one of the cool, popular kids, and I was a nerd. The laws and protocols of the schoolyard dictated that I keep my distance. It wasn't until we found ourselves studying the same communications degree at university that I realised she wasn't nearly as scary as I had thought at school, and we became friends. Since then, our lives have progressed in parallel. We both climbed the corporate ladder at the same pace; she specialised in marketing, and I went into public relations and then management consulting. We both deluded ourselves for the first ten years of our careers that we were indispensable at work and that what we were doing was terribly important. Then, about a year ago, we both realised we were over the corporate world and had lost our 'give-a-shit'. This was where our paths diverged a little bit. I dealt with my existential crisis by getting a part-time job so I could have time to write about it, while Emma medicated her meaninglessness with vodka shots and repeat doses of buff younger men. Then her party-girl lifestyle caught up with her and she was but a bee's dick away from contracting cervical cancer. Fortunately, Emma didn't develop cancer. She had contracted a virus that had caused pre-cancer cells on her cervix. Dr Lucy found them and surgically removed them before they turned into cancer.

When I tell Emma about my ovaries and imminent surgery, she tells me exactly what I need to hear. Having been under Dr Lucy's knife before, she assures me with authority that I'll be fine. Then she says, 'Far out, we're all turning to shit. It's depressing, isn't it? It's like we hit 30 and it's all downhill.'

A week and a day surgery later (the surgery was a stunning success, thank you for asking), I'm back in Dr Lucy's office to get the results from my operation. 'You have severe endometriosis,' she says. 'It was all over your left ovary, and in your fallopian tubes. You must have been in a lot of pain each month from your period.'

I shake my head. I hardly have any pain at all, I tell her. I get moody and bloated, but I don't get pain.

She shows me a picture of female reproductive organs covered in endometriosis. It looks disgusting, like an infestation of blood-sucking leeches. 'I have that inside me?' I say, horrified.

'Not any more,' Dr Lucy says. 'I cut it out. If it makes you feel better, it's also known as chocolate cysts.' Great. Just when I most need chocolate, Dr Lucy has to go and ruin it with horrible associations.

During the surgery, Dr Lucy removed almost half of my left ovary. In a nutshell, my right ovary is producing rubbish eggs, my left ovary has been chopped up and my fallopian tubes are blocked. 'Does any of this matter if I'm not in any pain?' I ask.

'It does if you want to have a baby,' Dr Lucy says. 'Your condition is very serious and it will only get worse. Are you planning on having a family?' she asks.

'No . . . I mean yes . . . I mean no. I don't know,' I say. 'I'm keeping my options open in case I want one some time in the future.'

'You don't have any more time,' Dr Lucy says in a tone that makes me shudder. 'You may already be unable to have a baby, but in 12 months it will almost certainly be too late: you will be infertile.'

As an expert in infertility treatment, she gives me a speech about how she sees women every day who are unable to have children because they waited too long and are simply too old to conceive.

'But I'm only 32,' I say. 'Surely that's not old.'

'It is in fertility years.'

Who knew that fertility years were like dog years?

She recommends that I go straight onto IVF because I don't have time to waste trying to conceive naturally. Given my blocked tubes and dud eggs, it's unlikely I'll be able to conceive the old-fashioned way anyway. Dr Lucy also tells me to start taking folic acid tablets and instructs me to go away, have a hard think and come back when I decide to try for a baby.

'That would be "if" rather than "when",' I say.

Dr Lucy gives me a half-smile as if to say, 'Want to bet on it?'

I leave Dr Lucy's office in a foul mood. How could nature insult me like this? How dare my ovaries box me into a corner and tell me that as far as fertility is concerned I'm pushing a Zimmer frame? I'm scandalised and outraged that my body is forcing me to make a decision before my brain is ready. Who do my ageing ovaries think they are to interfere in my life's plan like this?

It's not until I'm on the second-last square of my family-sized block of Cadbury's – who cares about dimply skin at times like this, and I've repressed Dr Lucy's comparison with the endometriosis – that I realise my life has changed for ever. Well, at least my perspective on my life has changed.

Until this moment, I had wholeheartedly believed that my life was filled with endless possibilities. I could do anything or be anyone I wanted – or so I thought. I tried not to worry too much about the decisions I made in my life, because if things didn't work out or if I changed my mind I could always do a U-turn and pick a new path to follow. I've lived a lot of my life like this. I've worked on five continents, lived in more homes than I can remember and had more lovers than

I'd want my mother to read about in this book. But, up until this point, I've always been pretty much in control of the timeline. Other than a couple of broken hearts and being retrenched from a job, I've been the one to decide what I want in my life and when I want to do it. But now my ovaries are waving their walking frame at me and taking delight in the fact that one of those 'cocky young people today who think they know everything' has fallen on her face.

I don't want to change my life just yet. I live in a tiny-yet-cosy apartment with my partner Chris and my neurotic poodle Toffee. I work part-time as a management consultant, flattering large companies into thinking that they actually control their employees, while spending the other part of my time pursuing my passion for writing. I have a handful of friends who mean the world to me, a pair of red tap shoes that come a close second and an agreement with Chris that we will discuss the baby question in 12 months' time and not a moment sooner.

Looks like I'm about to break that agreement.

# 2

# BLOODY CATHOLICS

Chris phones me after my doctor's appointment to ask about my test results. I tell him that there's no need to worry, because Dr Lucy removed all the endometriosis. Telling him what this might mean for the both of us can wait until tonight. Dr Lucy's words, 'It may already be too late,' reverberate through my brain, and I feel sick at the thought of having to give Chris the bad news.

Chris and I met via an Internet dating website. I did a search for educated single men who lived in a 15-km radius from my home, with no children, who didn't smoke, had left-wing politics and liked pets. A very short list of men met my criteria, so I systematically worked through it until I came to Chris. On our first date, Chris told me that he suspected most of his previous dates had been shopping for a husband and a father. He was a little offended that the women seemed more interested in the quality and viability of his sperm than in him.

I made it perfectly clear at the time that if he was in the market for a wife and a mother he should go to another store. I was pretty sure that an X-ray would prove that I didn't have a single maternal bone in my body. As for marriage, my parents' recent divorce was still a weeping sore for me, as was the revelation that neither of them had ever loved the other. What a waste of 32 years. I'd concluded that marriage was an antiquated institution that set people up for failure.

People only endured it until the pain of failure, social disapproval and dividing the assets seemed easier than having to put up with each other for another day.

Consequently, the baby subject had only been raised once. I'd been away for a week and a half at a meditation course and had missed Chris terribly. When I saw him I was intending to tell him how much I'd missed him, but without warning or any conscious forethought the words 'I want to have a baby' popped out of my mouth instead.

'I don't know where that came from,' I said. 'I swear, I have no idea why I just said that.'

Chris smiled knowingly. 'I'm not surprised,' he said. 'You're so maternal. You're maternal with Toffee, with your family, with your friends. The only one who doesn't see it is you. Maybe you needed ten days of reflection to work out what the rest of us already knew.' And then he said, 'You'd make a great mother.'

It was the first time anybody had ever said that to me. I've been told that I'd make a great manager, or a great writer, or that I can make a great curry. The concept of me being a great mother seemed like a category error, like an Amish computer technician or a sexy Conservative politician – it seemed like a misuse of language. I thought Chris must have been talking about somebody else. Nonetheless, I was surprisingly touched by the compliment. I felt my eyes well with tears and quickly looked away so Chris wouldn't see them. When I'd regained my composure, I said, 'I thought you didn't want kids.'

'I'm open to having kids,' Chris said. 'I just thought you didn't want them. And if I have to choose between having you and having kids, I choose you.'

At the time I found those words comforting. But now I'm not so sure. When he said that he wanted me more than he wanted kids, we were talking hypothetically. One week ago it was a matter of whether or not I wanted them, rather than whether or not I was able to have them. What if Chris is secretly or even subconsciously anticipating that in time I will lose my ambivalence and decide to have a baby? If

I can't have a baby and the decision has been taken out of our hands, will he start to view me as a mistake and not worth the sacrifice of being childless?

Walking home from work with these thoughts running through my head like a Lady Gaga song that just won't go away, I'm astounded by how many women are pushing prams. Where did these women come from? Was there a baby boom nine months ago and somebody forgot to send me the memo? How strange that I've never noticed them before. I always walk the same way home from work at roughly the same time, yet I've never before seen so many mothers and babies. In fact, before today I can't recall ever noticing them at all. They're everywhere: on the footpaths, in the cafes, in the park – all these women who were able to give their partner a child and all these babies who turned a couple into a family. I feel like they're swarming around me, closing in on me, taunting me and my corroded ovaries. They're like a plague of locusts.

When Chris comes home from work, I'm sitting on the couch waiting for him. The bottle of wine I opened 15 minutes ago is half empty. Chris greets me with raised eyebrows. It's unusual for me to hoe into a bottle of wine on my own.

'Good thing I'm not pregnant,' I say, topping up my glass.

Chris is the most grounded, well-balanced person I know. To be honest, it sometimes drives me crazy that he is always so calm and optimistic. Nothing fazes him. In the 12 months that I've known him, I've not once seen him lose his temper, worry and stress unnecessarily about something in the future, or ruminate about the past. That's not to say he's devoid of emotion or passion or conviction. Quite the contrary. I guess the best way to describe it is to say that he's a grown-up. He is just as grown-up as ever when I deliver my news.

'Can you love a barren woman?' I ask.

Putting his arm around me, Chris assures me that he will love me no matter what happens. I try to believe him but struggle with the idea. My insecurities are in a pitched contest with my self-worth, and my insecurities are dominating with a one–nil lead. I'm surprised how the prospect of infertility has rocked my confidence.

After listening to me talk around in circles for a couple of hours, Chris announces that he'd like to try for a baby. 'What? Just like that?' I ask in disbelief. 'You don't need any time to think about it, to weigh up the options, talk it over?' He shakes his head. 'You may not need time to think about it, but I do,' I say.

I can't understand Chris's certainty, but I envy it. This is the most serious decision I've ever had to make, and probably will ever have to make, in my life. I don't know how I can possibly make such an important decision so quickly. My ambivalence and doubt are amplified by my looming fertility expiry date.

Chris assures me that he'll be happy with whatever I decide. The only thing he feels strongly about is IVF. Chris is adamant that he wants to conceive the child naturally and doesn't want to use IVF. I tell Chris that Dr Lucy said my chances of conceiving naturally are between really bad and none, but Chris doesn't see it that way. He says we won't know if we can conceive naturally until we try.

One of Chris's primary reasons for refusing to use IVF is concern for my mental health. I've been battling with the black dog of my depression for many years. When it first started, my black dog had the upper paw. During my dark years, I had bouts of depression that would suck out every ounce of joy, hope and humour in my being, trample on it and then kick it into the gutter. And I would watch it rot in the gutter as I lay on the couch drinking gin, a broken soulless mess.

Thanks to a couple of years of therapy, some good drugs and Vipassana meditation, I've learned to tame my black dog, and even though I sometimes catch him lurking in the background of my life, I no longer let him overpower me. Chris is worried that I won't be able to cope with the emotional and financial stress of IVF, let alone all the artificial hormones, which, if the stories are to be believed, can turn the sanest woman into a mental case. He says IVF is a bit like gambling. People keep going back time and time again, each time clinging to the hope that this time will be different, this time they will get lucky. He probably has a point: for some people the odds are so low they'd have almost as much chance of hitting the jackpot at a casino as getting a baby.

Chris doesn't say so, but I wonder if there is more to his objection to IVF than just concern for my welfare. Is it also grounded in his religion? Chris is Catholic, and while he is the most liberal and open-minded Catholic I know, surely deep down he can't outrun his upbringing. Fucking Catholics, you can't win with them. First, they won't even allow contraception because life – and therefore sperm – is sacred. Then when you can't have kids, they turn around and won't allow technological intervention to alter God's so-called will. I mean, if God hadn't meant us to have IVF, then why did he give us electron microscopes, IVF clinics and smart doctors?

Chris and I have never had an argument. I think this is partly because neither of us has a particularly fiery temper, but I also think it's because we've never really had anything to disagree about . . . until now. Chris's stand on IVF really surprises me, and I feel backed into a corner. He says he wants to have a baby with me, but if I can't conceive naturally then he is essentially taking the decision out of my hands. By saying no to IVF, he could be saying no to having a baby.

I'm pissed off, but I don't share this with Chris because at the same time I also feel an odd sense of relief about his firm stance on IVF. I have to confess that I'm relieved because deep down I want to defer to somebody else. I want someone else to decide whether or not I have a baby, because if it turns out to be the wrong decision then it'll be somebody else's fault. I know this is neurotic and bordering on victim mentality, and completely unfair to Chris, but it's what I feel. If I end up regretting not having a baby for the rest of my life, I'd prefer to blame somebody else instead of myself.

# 3

# CLICK HERE FOR SPERM

As I lie awake in bed replaying the day's events, I'm overcome by a sense of love and gratitude for Chris. Despite not seeing eye to eye about IVF, he handled the news about my infertility like an absolute champion. Some men would have been secretly sizing up their suitcases, wondering how they could leave without making a scene if they came home to a half-sloshed girlfriend with a now-or-never ultimatum.

I roll over and wrap my arm around him. Chris is asleep, yet he instinctively grabs my hand and pulls me in closer. Even though we've only been together for a year, I'm in no doubt that he would be a great father. Out of all the men I have ever met, if I were to have children, I would want them to be with him. But what would I do if I didn't have Chris, or if he didn't want children? How would I feel if I was shacked up with Mr Good-Enough-For-Now, someone who is fun to play with at this moment in time but who has a very clear expiry date, or somebody who simply isn't father material? I'd have two decisions to make. Do I want kids? And do I want them enough to have them with Mr Inappropriate or on my own? If I decided to do it on my own, I'd also have to think about sourcing a father – or some sperm.

A couple of days later, my friend Lynn invites me to a dinner party. Lynn is a 40-something marketing executive with an infectious sense of serenity and a gorgeous cat called Woody. We met during a Vipassana meditation course.

Essentially the meditation course is ten days of hell where you and a roomful of strangers sit still and meditate for sixteen hours a day. Speaking isn't permitted, and you're not even allowed to make eye contact with anybody else. There is also no food permitted after midday. By making these sacrifices, you get to relive everything bad that's ever happened to you. I'm really selling it to you, aren't I? On the upside, you go home feeling the most unbelievable sense of peace, freedom and inner wisdom.

Lynn has also invited four other women from the Vipassana course. Having dinner with a group of people who willingly subject themselves to the kind of physical and mental rigour involved in Vipassana meditation is, shall we say, interesting. If your idea of a dinner party is great discussions about the latest books and films, sophisticated and witty conversations about pressing political and social issues, accompanied by wine and fine food, then you've clearly never been to a dinner party hosted by people who've studied Vipassana meditation.

We spend the first hour sitting on the floor of Lynn's house in silence with our eyes closed, meditating. While I understand the principles of Vipassana and know its benefits, I struggle to take this meditation session seriously. You have to admit that being invited over to somebody's house only to sit on the floor and not look at them or speak to them is pretty weird. Instead of being asked to bring our own drinks, we are asked to bring our own meditation cushion. I feel like I'm four years old again and having an afternoon nap at nursery. When I think nobody is looking, I sneakily half open my eyes to take a peek around the room. It occurs to me that even though I recently spent ten days and nights with these women, I barely know anything about them, because, well, we spent most of our time together sitting on the floor in silent meditation with our eyes shut. I start to wonder if the rest of the dinner party will be as weird and freaky as the beginning.

Once the meditation is over and the conversation begins to flow, I get my answer.

Almost immediately, the conversation veers towards babies and fertility. I don't know about you, but I don't usually get into deep conversations about fertility over dinner with people I don't really know. I suppose that when you've bonded, even silently, at a Vipassana retreat you can expect a whole lot more than the usual conversation about the latest books and films.

Two of us are in our 30s, and four are in their 40s. All of them except me are single. And all of them except me are certain they want a baby, or have gone through periods in the past when they have wanted one. Why do I suddenly feel that I've been sucked through a time–space wormhole and ended up on the set of a sitcom with a social message?

Our host, Lynn, would dearly love a child, but she believes a child should have a mother and a father and won't bring a child into the world unless she is in a stable relationship. Underneath her calm and philosophical exterior, I catch an unmistakable sadness in her voice as she talks of her fears that her time has run out and she will never be a mother. But Lynn also talks of a bigger picture. 'I may not have children myself, but I do have children in my life,' she says. 'It is different, as I get to care and have no direct responsibility, but I do feel fortunate that I can contribute to the lives of children as an aunt, god mum and "auntie" to friends' children.'

Fleur, a 40-something sculptor, shares the same view as Lynn. She oozes maternal energy. 'I always felt that I did want kids,' Fleur says, 'but I've never been in a relationship where I saw a future.' A few years ago, Fleur's sister-in-law offered to donate one of her eggs to Fleur. At the time, Fleur was already in her 40s and worried that her eggs were too old to conceive a baby. 'I was in tears,' she says. 'I've never been so moved.' Fleur thought about the offer briefly, because at the time her desire to have a child was quite strong. She did some research into the process her sister-in-law would go through if she were to donate her eggs, but they never spoke about it again. 'Deep down, I still have a fantasy of having a baby, but I only want kids if I'm in a relationship.' When it came to the time to make a decision, Fleur realised that her definition of family was more conservative than she'd thought it was.

27

The three other women don't see being single as an obstacle to having a baby. Kerry the management consultant and Linda the CEO of a manufacturing company are pregnant from donor sperm, and Mary the accountant is about to start IVF, using donor sperm as well. When I say they're using donor sperm, I don't mean they found some guy in a bar. Mary bought sperm from a local sperm bank via her IVF clinic. But she's quick to point out that when it comes to local sperm, it's slim pickings. She chose the best of the bunch but is still counting on the strength of her own genes when it comes to the appearance and intelligence of her child. Kerry and Linda reveal that they went further afield for their sperm and imported it from the US and Canada respectively.

And this is when the night becomes even weirder. They tell me that you can buy sperm on the Internet. Yep, you read it right – the Internet! I can't believe what I'm hearing. Who knew you could buy sperm online? If nothing else, it gives a completely new meaning to an 'Internet sex site'. How could I not know about this? Is there a department on Amazon or a category on eBay that I don't know about? Do the dodgy vendors who sell the dodgy Viagra and penis pumps throw it in for free instead of the standard set of steak knives? Maybe you really can buy anything on the Internet these days. 'So how does it work?' I ask naively. 'Do you bid for it on eBay?'

It turns out to be a little more complex than eBay but just as user-friendly. It's not an auction, but some sperm websites are open markets in so far as different sperm commands different prices depending on demand. For example, sperm from a tall, white, educated fireman who plays a musical instrument costs more than that of a short, bald, tone-deaf used-car salesman. Linda was able to see a photo of her donor, but in many cases photos are not available, so there's no way of knowing whether or not your tall, white, educated, musical fireman has a face like he ran into the back of his fire engine. Kerry's donor didn't have a recent photo of himself, but he specified that his celebrity likeness is Christian Slater.

There is something about putting a price tag on human

characteristics that I find offensive. Capitalism really does make all that is holy profane, as Karl Marx observed. Then, again, Marx had eight kids – including one with the housekeeper – so he obviously didn't face the same issues as a bunch of single women with a penchant for meditation.

The unit of measure for purchasing sperm is called a 'straw'. The regulations vary depending on where you live, but in general the sperm can be shipped direct to your door or doctor's office (turkey baster not included), or to your IVF clinic.

I look around the table at these women with a sense of bewilderment. I can't understand why they would buy sperm. They are all attractive, lively and intelligent. Surely men would be lining up to partner them. I jump to the conclusion that Linda is an ambitious career woman who cares more about her professional status than her relationship status, and Kerry and Mary are simply man-haters. But as the conversation moves on, I feel ashamed of the judgements I've just made. I like to think of myself as being an open-minded person, but yet again I am proved wrong.

Linda announces that she'd dearly love to be in a partnership. 'I seem like a stereotype,' she says. 'I'm the career woman leaving motherhood too late. But people get the cause and effect around the wrong way. I became successful at my career because my relationship broke up and I didn't have children, so that's where I channelled my energy.'

Linda was in a 13-year-long relationship that broke up around the time they would have started a family. 'My partner left me at 30,' she says. 'It took me five years to recover, and then I spent the next four years looking for a partnership. I had been thinking about children for a while, but I always thought that a man had to come first and a baby came second. Then I did Vipassana and realised that it was the other way around. I wanted a baby more than I wanted a man, so I decided I should do it myself. That's what Vipassana did. It silenced my thoughts and allowed me to hear my heart.'

Mary and Kerry tell similar stories. Both of them searched for partners, but as time ticked by and finding Mr Right in time became less and less likely, they decided to do it on their own. Kerry says that a big issue for her was letting go of the fantasy of the white picket fence and realising that having kids on her own didn't mean she'd be single for ever.

I don't know if it's all the baby hormones or the IVF drugs, but they all seem so calm and 'together'. Choosing to be a single mother seems so brave to me. Linda says that deciding to be a mother by choice was like her decision to run marathons. 'Initially I thought a half-marathon would be too hard, until I did it,' she says. 'Then I thought a full marathon would be too hard, but now I do them. Why should I think that I can't stretch my capabilities to be a mother on my own?' And Mary says, 'I knew I would have regrets if I didn't explore my options. I didn't want to be on my deathbed knowing that I didn't take control and take action.'

Kerry was nervous in the beginning because she was expecting a lot of judgement. But so far she hasn't got any. 'I thought I was going to offend people because it's so unconventional.' She didn't know what to expect when she announced her pregnancy at a family dinner party. 'I said, "I've got some news you're not expecting."' Her mum jumped in and said, 'You're engaged.' She guessed again: 'You're married.' Kerry said, 'No, I'm pregnant.' And her mother said, 'How?' The next day her parents sent flowers to work with a card saying: 'We can't wipe the smile off our faces.'

Mary's family were also supportive, her brother telling her to 'give it a crack'. But she has lost one friend over it. 'When I told him about my plans, he said that what I was doing was wrong and selfish. We haven't spoken to each other since.'

It's only now as I contemplate my own fertility that I realise that having a child is entirely selfish whether you have a partner or not. As I decide whether or not to have a baby, I am only thinking about how a baby will affect *my* life, *my* career, *my* relationships and *my* body. I'm not thinking about the impact on the child or on society or on the world. I'm not thinking about climate change or overpopulation and whether or not the world can cope with another mouth to feed. If I was thinking like that, my decision would be obvious. But because I'm being 'selfish', my decision is not at all obvious.

No matter what a woman decides when it comes to babies, she can be accused of being selfish: women who don't have children are selfish, single mothers are selfish, so are those who only have one child, as well as those who are seen to have too many.

Singling out women like Kerry and Linda seems unjustifiably critical. Although, that said, despite my respect and admiration for their courage, I secretly worry that they may be creating a minefield of problems in the future. How will they deal with the inevitable questions about daddy? Will the child be satisfied knowing that daddy was a fireman with a degree in Renaissance chamber music and brilliant aim when it came to wanking into a plastic sample jar? Will junior be placated with the knowledge that mummy invested in top-shelf sperm rather than settling for the cheapest she could find? But I suppose children have been dealing with this issue for centuries. Is it any different having an anonymous father from the Internet instead of one from a drunken one-night stand?

As the women talk through the options, I recall watching a documentary a couple of years ago about sperm donors. The film-makers asked the children, who were now teenagers, how they felt about their mother's decision. It surprised me that so many of the children interviewed were angry about not having a relationship with their fathers. Rather than focusing on the fact that their mother wanted them so much that she went to extraordinary lengths to have them, they focused instead on the father they will never have.

I remember one girl whose mother had bought the sperm from a sperm bank said, 'I'll probably never get to meet my father, but I just hope that he thinks about me.' The futility of her hope was heartbreaking. As if her father thinks about her. He probably doesn't even know she exists. The dichotomy in the perceptions of the daughter and donor was tragic – to the girl the donor was her dad, but to the donor she was most likely a wank that paid for a crate of beer or some outstanding bills. Some of my mates at university regularly donated sperm, and I am quite certain that in their minds they were not fathering children. All they were doing was earning some easy money, and they probably had forgotten all about it by the time they pulled up their pants and washed their hands.

Despite the potential problems associated with conceiving a child with donor sperm, I can't judge these women. How can I judge them when I'm lucky enough to have my own private sperm bank waiting for me at home? And I really do believe a lot of it is luck. Women are under so much cultural and economic pressure to delay motherhood that for many of us there is a window of only a few years when we are able to have children. If we don't happen to have a partner at that time, we're screwed. Well, technically, we're not screwed . . . you know what I mean.

Delaying motherhood is not the straightforward choice it's sometimes made out to be. The costs of housing and education and a hyper-competitive work culture mean that people feel compelled to delay children until they're financially secure. The consequence of these pressures is that young women spend their most fertile years focusing on establishing their careers and climbing the corporate ladder. In fact, if we don't establish ourselves professionally before we have babies, there's a good chance we'll end up living on Struggle Street. Imagine having a baby when we are biologically supposed to. We'd most likely still be in debt up to our eyeballs from our education and housing. And having just started out in our careers, our pay cheques would be pretty lousy. So we'd be taking time off work to have our baby when we had little or no savings, and when we returned to work we'd most likely be relegated to the 'mummy track', where our careers would progress slower and we'd earn less money than our childless sisters. Then when you consider that almost half of marriages fail, many of us would end up as poor single mothers with dead-end jobs. A happy thought indeed.

It's sad that our biology is so far out of sync with the cultural and economic realities of our work lives. No matter how much we judge 'selfish career women' for delaying motherhood and then having to go it alone, the realities of this imbalance don't change. For these women at the dinner party, like so many others, 'acquiring' sperm is their last and only option. To go to the effort of buying sperm means that they really, really want a child. Surely that counts for something.

As soon as I get home from the dinner party, I jump onto the Internet to check out the sperm website. The first thing I notice is that many of the donors are either in the military or Christian. I hit the jackpot when I stumble across a man who is both. According to his profile, he's a God-fearing poet who is trained in interrogation techniques and has served in the Middle East. What a catch! But this is not nearly as fascinating as the email I receive from the sperm bank a couple of days later. The email lists all the sperm that is on special offer this month. That's right: there are monthly discount sales on sperm. It's hard to fathom who would be motivated by a sperm sale. When *The Guardian* claims it costs in excess of £200,000 to raise a child, who would choose the father of their child based on the couple of hundred pounds they'd save on discounted sperm? I wonder how the donors feel about having their sperm discounted. I imagine it would be a rare man whose ego could withstand the indignity of the monthly sperm-sale email.

All this talk of and exposure to the world of online sperm makes me feel so old-fashioned. If I decide to have a baby, I'm going to try to do it with a penis.

# 4

# SPERM PARTY

The ticking of the biological clock has always been a torment reserved solely for women. If popular culture is anything to go by, women are kept awake at night by the sound of the ticking reverberating in their ears while their partners sleep soundly beside them. Men, it seems, can go on shagging and having kids for as long as they can get it up. Just look at Rupert Murdoch, Michael Douglas and Rod Stewart. And now, with the help of Viagra and pumps and whatever other meds and devices seem to turn up in my email inbox, men only hit their fertility use-by date when they keel over and die.

Medical doctor Sam Tormey disagrees. He talks about the 'Male Fertility Myth' and suggests that there is also a biological alarm clock on the man's side of the bed, even though most men are unaware of it. 'Who needs to listen to that pesky ticking when you have an impregnation apparatus that can be deployed at any time, with little more than a moment's notice, from puberty to the grave, or thereabouts?' Tormey says.

According to Tormey, male fertility problems are nearly as common as female ones, with almost half of all assisted-reproduction procedures being conducted because the man's swimmers are flailing around in the shallow end of the gene pool. It's not just a man's sperm count that drops with age; the little fellas can develop a whole range of problems. They can have misshapen heads or the wrong number of tails. Or they may not be strong enough to swim efficiently or, assuming that they can make it to the egg, to penetrate it when they get there. Sometimes the poor things simply get lost and are unable to find the egg at all. And sadly, guys, a GPS isn't going to fix this problem.

Motility issues are not the only problems for old-man sperm. As men get older, their sperm show signs of increased DNA damage, increasing the risk of health problems in the child. This has been linked with higher rates of miscarriage, congenital heart problems, dwarfism, lower IQs, Down's syndrome and autism.

'I have lost count of the number of 40-something dads who have poured out their anxieties to me that the MMR jab might result in autism in their toddler (exhaustive research proves that it doesn't), but I haven't yet had the courage to point out that they have already trebled or quintupled their child's risk of the disorder by "leaving it so late" to become a dad,' Tormey says.

Chris is only 34, so technically his swimmers should be strutting around in their speedos, preening themselves and limbering up for the big race. I'm only 32 and I could already be too old. What if Chris has underperforming sperm to match my substandard eggs? What if my own private sperm bank turns out to be as – ahem – liquid as Lehman Brothers? To rule out this possibility, I invest in a do-it-yourself sperm-testing kit I find on the Internet. You really can buy anything on the Internet. For the bargain price of thirty quid, the manufacturer promises that you can test the concentration of motile sperm in the privacy of your own home. It doesn't test all the other things, like shape and navigational abilities, but at least it will tell us something.

The test is a lot more complex than a pregnancy or ovulation test. There's no peeing on sticks for this test. Oh no: this test takes planning and probably a decent pass in high-school chemistry. This is a worry, because I dropped all my science subjects at school as soon as I was able. And should I be worried that the instructions are written in 'Chinglish'?

I tell my friend Jules about the test, which involves test tubes, a thermometer and a funnel, and she begs me to let her conduct it. 'I can bring a Bunsen burner,' she offers enthusiastically. A few hours later I'm telling my friend Brandy about the test and she is just as excited about participating in a science experiment as Jules.

What is it with lesbians and sperm? Or is it just lesbians and science experiments? Out of all of my friends, it is my two lesbian friends who insist on participating in the testing of Chris's sperm. Not wishing to offend either of them, I decide to host a dinner party in three days' time and turn the sperm testing into an event. From what we can glean from the instructions, we need to wait because Chris has to ejaculate and then abstain for three days for optimum test results.

A few hours later, Brandy phones back to express some concerns. Her colleague Patrick is horrified on Chris's behalf that we have planned a public sperm test. He told her that a sperm test is a very sensitive thing for a man and Chris is unlikely to want an audience, especially if the test results turn out to be bad. Patrick asked if we have Chris's permission.

It hasn't occurred to me that Chris would have any objection to having an audience. It's not as if we are all going to stand around and watch him wank. And as for his sperm count, I've been completely open with my friends and family about my shitty eggs, so I assumed Chris would be just as open about his sperm. The more I think about it, though, the more I can see that Patrick may have a point. I don't feel less of a woman because my eggs are dodgy, but in our culture a man with dodgy sperm is considered less virile and less masculine. I tell Brandy and Jules that the dinner party is on hold until I speak to Chris.

It turns out that Chris has not linked his identity to his sperm count, and he agrees to allow Jules and Brandy to test his sperm. Neither Chris nor I have very good attention to detail, so we are happy to outsource the test to our friends. I ask Chris again if he's sure he's OK with the sperm-testing dinner party. 'What will happen if your sperm count is low?' I ask.

'Then it's low, and we'll have to deal with that if and when it happens,' Chris says calmly.

The night of the dinner party, I'm feeling a little anxious. Actually, I'm feeling a lot anxious. I'm surprised by my reaction; I'm surprised that I really do care if Chris is fertile or not. I don't take my anxiety to mean that deep down I really do want kids; I think it's more about the loss of possibility. If we do decide to try for a baby, conceiving will be hard enough with my crappy eggs. I assume that if Chris has fertility problems as well, it really will be game over.

During the starter and the main course, the conversation mostly centres around the instructions for the sperm test and the equipment we'll need. Jules makes it quite clear that she is the lead scientist and Brandy is her lab assistant. Jules is taking her responsibilities so seriously it seems the only thing she is missing is a white coat.

After we finish eating, Chris excuses himself, saying, 'I suppose this will be the only time in my life when it will be socially acceptable to go off and have a wank in the middle of a dinner party.' I follow Chris into our bedroom to offer my oral . . . I mean moral, support, and we roll around the bed laughing at the absurdity of the situation. After about ten minutes, we compose ourselves and get down to business.

Chris and I emerge from the bedroom wishing that we'd stayed in there longer. This has nothing to do with fooling about in the bedroom. It turns out that in our absence Jules, Brandy and Brandy's partner Samantha have busied themselves cleaning our kitchen. In the time we've been away, they've scrubbed the stove and reorganised our cutlery drawer. If we'd taken time for a post-wank cuddle, who knows? Perhaps the girls would have cleaned our whole apartment.

Jules and Brandy take the sample from Chris and I feel oddly protective and territorial. It doesn't seem right for other women to be handling Chris's sperm, even though it's safely contained in a test tube and their interest in it is purely scientific. Having said that, though, the first time Brandy met Chris she said, 'You've done well there, babe. Bet he's got great sperm.' I had no idea at the time that less than 12 months later she would be testing her assertion.

Jules pours the sperm into a test tube and pretends to take a sip, saying, 'Delicious. So this is what I've been missing out on all these years.' When the laughter dies down, the girls get on with the business of testing – boiling, measuring, filtering. Then we have to wait for an hour to see what colour the sperm turns. There is a scale from bright purple to bright pink. The pinker the sperm turns, the better the result. We position the sperm sample so that it's a table centrepiece, not unlike a lava lamp, while we have dessert. As it slowly changes colour the conversation drifts onto other topics, but I struggle to keep up. I'm trying to play it cool, but I can't take my eyes off the test tube. I'm staring at it, secretly willing it to turn pink.

After a few minutes, the sperm turns purple and my stomach sinks. I check the colour chart and see that the shade of purple in the test tube corresponds with the infertile section of the chart. Chris senses my dismay and he says, 'It's only been a few minutes, puss cat. Let's just wait until it's time.'

It occurs to me that by turning into an anxious mess, I am putting more pressure on Chris. It's his sperm after all, so surely he has the most invested in the result. If the result is bad, I don't want to add to his disappointment by having him think that he's let me down. He didn't go to pieces when I told him about my dodgy eggs, so I have no right to be so selfish about his sperm. I set myself the challenge of not looking at the sperm until the end of the test.

I fail miserably, but eventually the alarm beeps on Jules's watch and it's time to read the results. Jules holds the sperm up to the colour scale and we all conclude that Chris has passed the test with flying colours – his sperm sample is as bright pink as the brightest colour square on the chart. Chris roars like a caveman, I breathe a sigh of relief, lead scientist Jules and her assistant Brandy congratulate each other on a job well done, and Samantha takes photos of us holding the test tube of sperm. A dinner party like this one deserves to be captured for posterity.

As the party comes to a close, Brandy asks, 'How do you know the test is accurate?'

Chris laughs. 'We don't. We may have just spent £30 and a couple of hours messing around with food dye.'

'If nothing else, this will probably be the only time I'll get to play around with sperm,' Jules says.

# 5

# JUST A MOTHER

The thing that scares me most about motherhood is the possibility of losing my identity. I genuinely believe that motherhood is a noble thing to do, but, despite this, I don't think I could handle being 'just' a mother. People strip mothers of their identity so readily that half the time they don't even know they're doing it. It's almost as if once a woman pops out a baby – or perhaps it's as soon as her pregnant belly becomes obvious – all she has been and all that she has accomplished beforehand is somehow cancelled out.

I'm reminded of my fear of losing my self at Scott's birthday party. Scott is a friend of Chris and he's an excellent introducer. He must have done one of those networking courses. When he introduces people, he doesn't just say their name, he also gives a little bit of information about the person so as to give context and start a conversation. At the party he introduces me to his other guests by saying, 'This is Kasey, Chris's partner. She's a management consultant and she's writing a book about how much she hates work.' But then he introduces me to a woman who has a baby strapped to the front of her. 'This is Melanie, Henry's mother.'

There's no doubt that Henry is absorbing the focus of the room, but the introduction still grates. Surely Melanie is more than 'just' Henry's mother. What did she do before she had Henry? What does she do now when she's not mothering Henry?

Later in the night, I ask Melanie how she feels about being introduced as just an extension of her child. She laughs and says it happens so often she doesn't notice any more. This is scarier still. Not only has Melanie lost her identity, she's become so desensitised to being viewed as 'just' a mother that she's now oblivious to it.

Melanie says she still felt like an individual when she was pregnant. People would want to know about her – how she was feeling physically, how she was feeling emotionally and whether or not she needed to sit down. That all changed as soon as she gave birth; nobody seems to give a damn any more. It's all about Henry.

I wouldn't dream of denying Henry the limelight. He's a gorgeous little boy deserving of lots of attention. I can also see how Melanie would be proud to be identified as Henry's mother. But why does she have to be only Henry's mother? Why can't she still be all the things she was before?

Melanie says that even in the privacy of her mothers' group, the women have reduced themselves to 'just' mothers. She's been attending her mothers' group for four months, but in that time all she has ever discussed with the other mothers is mothering and baby issues. 'I can give you intimate details about all of the mothers' cracked nipples and how well their babies sleep, but I couldn't tell you what they did before they had a baby, or what they're interested in or passionate about other than their kid.'

Melanie has met with these women for a couple of hours every week for four months. That's over 30 hours of conversation, and she knows nothing about them outside of their role as mothers. How can you form a meaningful relationship based on nipple condition and controlled crying?

I'm dismayed to hear about Melanie's mothers' group, but I'm not surprised. That's why parents are so goddamn boring and why there is a great divide between parents and non-parents. I've yet to meet a new parent who can speak of anything other than their child. I've seen it happen with some of my colleagues. Colleagues, both male and female, who were once great conversationalists – worldly, interesting and interested – are reduced to boring shells of their former selves. It amazes me how when people become parents they somehow lose their relevance filter. Their conversational repertoire is as extensive and repetitive as one of those toys that speaks when you pull the cord. 'Little Johnny slept for six hours straight last night.' Pull the cord. 'Little Johnny said "Dada" for the first time.' Pull the cord. 'Little Johnny slept for six hours last night.' But unlike those dolls with a ripcord, their human counterparts don't have batteries that can be removed in order to get a moment's peace. I've been caught in situations where the conversation of new parents is so mind-numbingly boring I can't even pretend to be interested. How can I possibly be expected to be interested in how many wet nappies little Johnny had yesterday? I can't tell you how much I don't care about an infant's excretions.

Not only are new parents boring as batshit, they're also super-competitive and judgemental of each other. (OK, OK, so that was a super-competitive, judgemental statement.) Leora Tanenbaum writes in *Catfight* that when women become mothers their whole identity becomes an extension of their child's. If you have a good child, then by extension you're a good mother, which is synonymous with being a good person. The flipside is that if your child is a little git, then so are you. It doesn't matter what you might have accomplished in your life up until that point or what your plans are for the future. The world views you as 'just' a mother and therefore judges your worth by your child. Your self-worth is based entirely on how beautiful, how clever or how well-behaved your child is compared with other children, and it becomes the only way you can assert your identity or demonstrate achievement. Even worse, this is why mothers are blamed for most of society's ills. Because women are usually charged with the primary responsibility for raising children, they are the ones blamed when things go pear-shaped and the cute, mischievous child grows up to be an adult-sized shit with a cocktail of impulse-control problems and anger-management issues.

Talking with Melanie, it dawns on me that if I have a baby, not only will the world forget that I'm a partner, a consultant and a writer and see me instead as 'just' a mother, I could quite possibly accept this redefinition of my identity and view myself this way too. And then, if my child turns out to be a psychopath, a megalomaniac or, worse, a Conservative voter, it'll be all my fault. No matter how successful I have been in other areas of my life, I will be judged by one criterion alone.

My fears that motherhood will cannibalise other aspects of my life aren't irrational, either. A 2009 study by Jessica Woodroffe called 'Not Having It All: How Motherhood Reduces Women's Pay and Employment Prospects' found that motherhood did indeed impact upon women's professional opportunities and identities. In fact, it even starts in pregnancy: 'Each year, an estimated 440,000 women miss out on pay or promotion as a result of pregnancy.' And then upon returning to work after maternity leave, 13 per cent of women had reduced seniority, 20 per cent had reduced responsibilities and almost a third of women felt their promotion prospects had been reduced.

Wouldn't it be nice to think that it's a choice, that mothers are in fact satisfied with their stagnant careers and low-level jobs because they are so fulfilled by motherhood. But even if we assume that mothers are fulfilled and enriched by mothering, it just doesn't make sense that they'd choose a low-level job, synonymous with low pay, low status and limited autonomy.

I find it very hard to believe that just as our bodies expel the placenta at birth, we would also rid ourselves of our need for achievement and recognition. Let's face it, professional success offers far more status in our society than success as a mother. Not only will motherhood strip me of my identity and make me a dinner-party bore, it will also limit my career prospects and my work satisfaction. I add another item to my mental pros and cons list for having a baby.

A couple of days later, I'm discussing this issue with my friend Jane and lamenting the unfairness and inequality. If we have a baby, Chris will get to keep his identity as a freelance journalist and a social commentator. He won't be introduced at parties as 'just' a father. In fact, rather than being reduced, his identity will be expanded. He will be a father and a journalist. Jane can't see why I'm making such a fuss. 'All I've ever wanted is to be a mother,' she says. 'I can't wait to be introduced at a party as my baby's mother.'

I envy Jane. Imagine knowing all your life that you're meant to be a mother. Maybe there is a motherhood gene that I just didn't get. In the days following my talk with Jane, I come across a newspaper report about a group of researchers who have found a motherhood gene in mice. It's called the Mest gene. Apparently, the mice mothers in the study who didn't have this gene were so negligent that they should have had the Department of Mice-Child Services on their tails. They didn't feed their babies or care for them in the same way as the mice that did have the gene. I'm not sure if we can extrapolate this study to humans – I haven't come across any studies on human Mest deficiency – but if there is a human Mest gene, then Jane definitely has it.

Jane and I grew up together. She recently married and is expecting their first child. She says that she always used to feel inadequate when we were younger and we'd talk about what we wanted to do when we grew up. I would bang on about all my big plans for saving the world when all she wanted to do was be a mother. This is a bit of a wake-up call to me. I haven't come close to saving the world; all I've ever done is work in big companies making money for people who already have enough. And in a few months' time, Jane will be the mother she always wanted to be.

Now it's my turn to feel inadequate.

# 6

# EMMA'S ULTIMATUM

'I don't think my little sister was supposed to happen,' Emma confides the next day after I tell her about my conversation with Jane. I am sitting on her couch eating a bowl of ice cream because it's the only human food she has in the house. There is plenty of dog food, dog bones and dried pigs' ears in the cupboards; Emma's dogs never go without. 'I suspect Mum manipulated that situation with my sister,' Emma says. 'Dad got fixed after that because Mum couldn't be trusted.'

If there is a motherhood gene, Emma is quite certain that that particular number didn't come up in her genetic lottery. She's even less likely to have kids than I am. Her mother, Jenny, despairs at this. Jenny is baby crazy. Emma claims that her mum would have had five kids if her dad hadn't had the snip.

Emma's utter lack of interest in motherhood has been a source of friction between her and Jenny for as long as she can remember. A couple of years ago at a family gathering, Emma's aunt Hilde asked if she was going to have kids. When Emma said she didn't think so, her mum said, 'That'll teach me for raising an independent woman. If only I'd known at the time that it would mean I wouldn't get any grandkids.'

Jenny may yet get her wish, because, like me, in the past week Emma has also been forced to face the baby question. Unlike me,

47

though, it's not her biology that has backed her into a corner. Rather, it's her boyfriend, Matt.

Matt, along with Emma's health scare, signalled the end of her experimental phase. Rather than discarding Matt after a couple of weeks of fun, like all the other boys, Emma quite liked him and decided to keep him around. Almost a year later, they are still going strong. It is unexpected when Matt sits Emma down to deliver his ultimatum. It's the conversation that so many of our girlfriends have agonised over. Should they have it? When should they have it? Where should they have it? Only this time it's in reverse. It's Matt who is the one saying that he wants a family and he doesn't have time to waste with somebody who doesn't want the same thing. He tells Emma that if she's not prepared to start a family within the next 18 months then they should break up now.

Emma admits that she's a little offended by the ultimatum. 'I expected he'd bring it up sooner or later and can understand where he's coming from,' she says. 'But it hurts that he implied being with me is wasting time if I don't produce children.'

There really is no justice when it comes to making babies. The women at the meditation dinner party the other night would have loved to have the conversation that Matt and Emma are having. Emma, on the other hand, is nursing a bruised ego at the realisation that she's not enough on her own and that Matt doesn't want her unconditionally. It seems completely legitimate for Emma to be offended by the ultimatum, yet it's never occurred to me before that this may also be how men feel when their girlfriends raise the now-or-never conversation.

When my friend Narelle had the baby talk with her boyfriend of two years I remember saying to her, 'If he doesn't love you enough to have kids with you, then kick him to the kerb, girlfriend. Move on and find somebody who does.' I didn't spend a single moment thinking about how her boyfriend might feel. It's possible that he too would have been hurt that Narelle's love for him was conditional. It's only now that I realise that when it comes to long-term relationships, love is perhaps secondary or, at best, equal to the practical considerations. It's about whether or not the couple share the same life vision, and, sadly, this is yet another example of how love does not conquer all. I fear that my relationship with Chris has also just entered the land of practical considerations. Chris has made it clear that he wants a baby, even though he assures me that he'll be happy with whatever I decide. But for how long, I wonder. He might be happy not to have children this month, or maybe even next month. What if he changes his mind the month after that and I haven't? It's possible that the baby question is like a terminal disease in our relationship. It will fester just below the surface until one day the immune system of our relationship can no longer suppress it and Chris will deliver the same ultimatum to me that Matt has given to Emma.

Despite her hurt feelings, Emma respects Matt for being upfront with her. 'This is not something we can compromise on, so it's good to get it out in the open.'

Concerned that Emma might be being talked into motherhood against her deeper instincts, I tell her about a book I've started reading to work out what I feel about this whole motherhood thing, now that my body has handed me an ultimatum. The book's called *Do I Want to Be a Mom?* by Diana L. Dell and Suzan Erem. Darcey, a woman interviewed in the book, says, 'I'm not the kind of woman who gets talked into things, but there I was, pregnant, wanting the baby, but not sure I wanted to be a mom. He had told me that some day I would want a child. I talked myself into it. But in the end, I had to face the truth; I did it for him and for the sake of the marriage, and I knew those were two lousy reasons.'

Emma assures me that she won't have a baby just to please Matt. 'I don't think I'd agree to it if I really didn't want to do it,' she says. 'I don't think I've ever really done anything to please anybody else – except pleasing my parents when I was younger, but even then that was just so I didn't get grounded. It comes back to my fundamental selfishness.'

Emma told Matt during the ultimatum conversation that she needed time to think about it. But she knew immediately that their relationship had changed for ever. 'There's no more playtime,' she says. 'These are very grown-up conversations and it really hit home that I've reached a phase in my life where I need to make grown-up decisions.'

'What's your gut telling you?' I ask.

'I don't want to have a kid because I know it's going to be hard,' Emma says. 'I don't like doing things that are hard. And I just know I'd end up having a little shit.'

After dissecting Emma's dilemma, I share my news with her. Chris has just landed a new job teaching journalism at a university. When I first met Chris he was working part-time as an editor so he could spend the rest of his time working as a freelance journalist. He really enjoys the freedom and autonomy of freelancing, so I'm surprised that he wants to re-enter the world of full-time employment. But he's hoping that as an academic in the field of journalism he'll still get the opportunity to write for the media as well as having the added bonus of colleagues and job security.

I confide that my first thought when Chris told me the news was not about his job satisfaction. Instead, it was about the extra money and security that would come in handy if we have a baby. It popped into my head just like that.

Maybe I do have the Mest gene after all.

# 7

# A WHOLE LOT OF SHIT WITH A GLIMPSE OF BRILLIANCE

I need to get to the bottom of this motherhood business. I need someone who's had similar experiences to me – and who doesn't have a vested interest in me getting knocked up. I call my friend Sophie for a catch up. I met Sophie at a Women in Business networking function a few years ago. At the time, we shared the same ambition to climb the corporate ladder. She's currently on maternity leave with her second child and is looking forward to returning to the world of adult conversation, lunch breaks and personal grooming.

I was surprised when Sophie had a second baby, because I distinctly remember her telling me after she'd had her first that it was the biggest mistake of her life. She confides that she wrote in her diary, 'I will never, ever do this again. I can't believe I brought this upon myself.' She remembers watching one of the mothers at her mothers' group stare lovingly at her baby and thinking to herself at the time, 'Why don't I feel like that about my baby?'

I can only guess that she doesn't feel like that now, because, less than three years later, she has brought it upon herself again. When I question Sophie about why she had a second child when she found the first one so hard, she tells me that motherhood is 70 per cent monotonous, thankless hard work, 20 per cent OK and then there is 10 per cent that is pure delight and makes it all worth it. She must have been stuck in the 70 per cent when she sent me this email. I'm including all of it below because it's simply too revealing to leave anything out.

Lately I have noticed that I sit around at mothers' group and Tupperware parties watching the women who all seem so happy. With their life, with their kids, with their husbands. And I wonder, what is wrong with me? Why are they all so happy? An overwhelming sadness engulfs me.

I am a mouse in a mousetrap . . . Run, run, run.

Working 14 hours straight a day. Menial, hard, physically and emotionally draining work. Work, work, work.

6.30 a.m., hear baby stirring. Try to ignore him, hoping he will go back to sleep. 6.45, no such luck. Up, change him, feed him. Quickly, try and get the dishwasher unpacked and the breakfasts ready before the other one gets up. No such luck — 'Get out, get out, Daddy, I want Mummy,' yells the three year old. Throw a load of washing on. 'I don't want you, I don't want brekkie, throw it in the bin,' shortly follows from up the hallway. Feed solids to baby — spits Weetabix all over the table and me. 'I don't want brekkie,' yells the three year old. 'Throw it in the bin.' Go to throw his breakfast in the bin and he yells blue murder. Finally he starts to eat. Try to feed baby some pears. Coughs it all over me.

Stay calm, stay calm. Everything will stay calm if I stay calm.

8 a.m. and still have not managed a hot cup of tea or any breakfast for me. Clean up the food that covers the table. Wash the dishes. Empty the dishwasher. Wipe down bibs. Wipe down the kitchen bench. Put the washing out. Fold yesterday's clean washing. Peel some veggies to steam for the baby. Cook veggies, purée veggies, clean up kitchen, stack dishwasher. Do a batch of ironing.

9 a.m., manage to down a cool cup of tea and eat some cold Weetabix. Better put baby to sleep. Maybe I could put Play School on for an hour so I can sit down and relax. No such luck. If I vacuum now, I won't have to later. Play School on. Quickly vacuum, dust and put all the washing away. Baby nearly due up. Quick, better have a shower. No time to dry my hair today. Put on another load of washing.

Duck out before lunch to get something for dinner. Quick, we'd best get back in time for baby's lunch. Prepare lunch. 'I don't want lunch,' yells the three year old. 'Throw it in the bin.' Go to throw his lunch in the bin and he yells blue murder. Finally he starts to eat. Try to feed baby lunch. He eats pretty well and then starts to cough it all over me. Clean up the food that covers the table. Wash the dishes. Empty the dishwasher. Wipe down bibs. Wipe down the kitchen bench. Bring the washing in and put out another load. Three year old has been whingeing and whining most of the morning. 'I want this, I want that, I don't want this, I don't want that. It is black, no, it is white.'

Stay calm, stay calm. Everything will stay calm if I stay calm.

Must be time for a break. Children in bed. 'I don't want to sleep,' yells the three year old. I don't care. Maybe I could sit down for a while. Going out this afternoon, though, so best get dinner ready instead. Sit down with a cup of tea. Pick up toddler book to work out how to manage the trying toddler. Pick up baby book to work out why he would be waking up at night. Any time left? Half an hour maybe. Pick up Buddhism for Young Mothers. Read a paragraph and fall asleep for 15 minutes.

2.15 p.m., hear the baby stirring. Try to ignore him, hoping he will go back to sleep. No such luck. Up, change him, feed him. Bang Bang — three year old is kicking his legs against the wall beside his bed. Open the door and greet him with maniacal cheerfulness. 'Go away, Mummy, I don't want to go to shop/park/friend's place.' Bang goes the door as he slams it.

Stay calm, stay calm. Everything will stay calm if I stay calm.

Dress the baby, pack the nappy bag. Nappies, wipes, snacks, water. Three year old finally gets up. Doesn't want to wear the blue shoes, wants to wear the other blue shoes that no longer fit. Tantrum brewing . . . bang. Lose it. 'Oh for goodness' sake child you cannot wear those ones,' I shout, grabbing him roughly. 'Just put these on.' Three year old yells right back at me. He hits me and shouts. Roughly put him on the Quiet Chair. Good luck. Stay calm, stay calm. Everything will stay calm if I stay calm. GOD, how can I remain so incredibly, inhumanly patient? Finally calm down and manage to talk some sense into the child.

Finally ready to go. Everyone happy. Baby has a toy, three year old has food.

Out and about doing chores. Craving adult company so organise an hour of play with a friend. Manage some broken conversation in between trying to teach a three year old to share and baby not to eat bark.

Quickly, we'd best get back in time for dinner. Prepare dinner. 'I don't want dinner,' yells the three year old. 'Throw it in the bin.' Go to throw his dinner in the bin and he yells blue murder. Finally he starts to eat. Try to feed baby dinner. He eats pretty well and then starts to cough it all over me. Clean up the food that covers the table. Wash the dishes. Empty the dishwasher. Wipe down bibs. Wipe down the kitchen bench. Bring the washing in.

Nearly there, nearly there. Bath the baby. Think the three year old had a bath yesterday so don't bother today and just put him in his pyjamas. Put our dinner in the oven. Go through house putting away clothes and toys. Sweep the floor. Baby starting to whinge. Three year old watches TV. I feed the baby. Nearly there. Nearly there.

6.50 p.m., baby fed and in bed. I stand at the fridge with a sigh of relief as I realise it is nearly over and pour myself a cold, cold glass of wine. I take a sip. It is all OK.

Tidy up the kitchen, finish off dinner. Husband arrives home to a cheerful three year old. 'How was your day?' he asks innocently. I fill my glass again.

I sit down. Oh no — time for toilet and teeth and stories with the three year old. Lie in bed with three year old reading stories, feeling a warm glow. Is it the wine, the fact that I got through another day or the pure enjoyment of reading stories with my son?

Finally, children are in bed. Husband wants to debrief on his corporate day and I nod at the appropriate places. Get up, serve dinner, eat dinner, watch something mundane on television.

8.30 p.m., fighting off sleep. Time to fall into bed.

(One child or both may wake up calling for me in the middle of the night. Fall out of bed and stumble to their rooms quickly in case they wake the other. Quickly comfort child and stumble back to bed. Lie awake for an hour afterwards listening — praying for silence. Finally go back to sleep.)

6.30 a.m., hear baby stirring. Try to ignore him, hoping he will go back to sleep. 6.45, no such luck.

Hardest job in the world, I say. Such monotony, such routine. Thankless, hard work. But I can't complain, can I, because I am so lucky to have them. So lucky to have two healthy and beautiful children. I can't complain, can I? I have no right to complain, do I?

It can be so crappy, this phase of life. You give up everything. Your identity, your body, your appearance, your career. And all I really want is the feeling that what I have given up is appreciated. Appreciated by someone. But that just doesn't seem to come. I feel like I am being sucked dry.

I whinge and I complain and I feel so terribly sad at times at the state I see myself in, but then something will happen and I feel like I have no right to feel this way.

My husband struggles with the roller coaster that is me. But motherhood is a roller coaster. It's a whole lot of shit, and then glimpses of brilliance and light. My three year old just came in with his hat and a bucket on his head. 'Look, Mummy, I have two hats on.' And when I say it's time for a story, he says, 'I want the cuddle story,' and virtually strangles me with a cuddle. He'll hear a plane and go running out around the yard yelling, 'Mummy, Mummy, look, look . . . a plane. Quick, Mummy, look.' His grandfather pointed out a blue bike the other day and he corrects him: 'No, Poppie, it is aqua, not blue.' So much crap, but then things like this happen and you wonder why you should be complaining. My baby boy is a pure delight. He pants and jumps up and down when he sees me or his big brother. Yet I lost it this morning in the middle of trying to get things done because he would not go to sleep.

I don't know about you, but she's not really doing a good job of selling me on motherhood.

# 8

# THE FIVE-MINUTE FIX

Sophie tells me that if I want to know what motherhood is really like I should read *The Mask of Motherhood* by Susan Maushart. It takes almost two weeks to read the book, even though I make it my top priority. That's not a comment on Maushart's writing abilities. It takes so long to read the book because I have to put it down after every couple of pages to do some deep-breathing exercises. I'm on the verge of an anxiety attack every time I turn a page.

There are many things that distress me about Maushart's revelations on motherhood. Motherhood looks like a scene in a horror movie: a place of bleak deprivation and loss, a place from which there is no return. The worst of it by far are the bits about gender inequality. I worked out a long time ago that the 'anything boys can do, girls can do better' mantra of my youth was bullshit. We can't do it better because we are not allowed to do it better. If that sounds cynical, then why does the pay gap between men and women still exist – and why is it even worsening in some countries that claim to value equality? But I digress. Even though I know it's a man's world, I've always clung to the hope that equal opportunity is a realistic goal, albeit a long-term one.

According to Maushart, when a woman becomes a mother equal opportunity is as attainable as pain-free childbirth. You need look no further than the language we use for parenting. When a man 'fathers' a child, it takes about five minutes, feels great and he often gets to have a nap after it. When a woman 'mothers' a child, she's signing on for years of monotonous, back-breaking domestic work at the expense of her identity, autonomy and career, and she doesn't get to sleep for about ten years.

Then again, Maushart's book was first published in 1997. Surely things have changed in the intervening period, haven't they? I mean, we live in a time when, if a 2007 report from the BBC is to be believed, some men go through 'phantom pregnancies', including experiencing symptoms such as morning sickness, cramps, back pain and even swollen stomachs, when their partners are pregnant. Surely after experiencing his phantom pregnancy, he's rolling up his sleeves, fully prepared to do his share of the parenting and domestic work required in raising the child.

Not so fast. Along with those phantom pregnancies, research shows that the modern image of domestic equality is also something of a phantom. I'm gutted when I read about the countless studies from all over the developed world showing that the only thing that has changed since our grandmothers' time is our expectations. It seems that the realities of gender inequality in child-raising and domestic work have remained largely unchanged over the past 50 years. In fact, the biggest inequality is no longer between men and women; it's between mothers and everyone else.

This has got to be the worst outcome imaginable. Not only are we lumped with all the work and all the sacrifice, we also have to deal with the shock and dismay that our relationships are no more equal than our mothers' were, and that no matter how much our partner will rub our belly and talk to the foetus, when the baby's on the outside, he'll be conspicuously absent when it comes to changing nappies, sterilising bottles, washing laundry and puréeing food. And even if his participation is above average, he will never actually feel responsible. When (or if) he gets up in the night, we'll think he's doing us a favour rather than simply fulfilling his responsibility as a parent. We'll feel 'lucky' when we get a single night off in months to go out on our own. And all the mental work and planning involved in raising a child, such as scheduling medical check-ups, arranging babysitters or alternative childcare, making sure there are always nappies in the house and deciding when and how to start solids, will always be our responsibility. And, as always, it will also be our fault when something goes wrong.

A little voice inside me says, 'Yes, yes, but that's other women. It's not me.' Surely my experience of motherhood will be different. I'm a feminist and Chris has read more Germaine Greer, Susan Faludi and Adrienne Rich than I have. Just when I'm starting to convince myself, the following passage from Maushart's book sends me spiralling into despair:

> We delude ourselves that we will be different. We will buy our way out, we tell ourselves, with nannies and fast food and housekeepers. We will think our way out with positive affirmations of our own self-worth, or with child-rearing theories that promise to reveal 'the secrets of happy children' or 'the path to positive parenting' in ten easy lessons. We will love our way out, with revolutionary marriages and partnerships that promise liberty, equality and justice for all.

When my friend tells me that every woman who has a baby will be profoundly disappointed in her partner soon after the baby arrives, I just assume she is being overly bitter and cynical and that it says more about her own shitty marriage than gender issues in general. But after doing a little more research, I find that the statistics are on her side. If I haven't ruined your day already, here are some numbers that ought to depress you.

Maushart writes that after the birth of her first child, a woman's domestic workload increases by 91 per cent to an average of 55 hours and 48 minutes per week. Her partner's workload increases zero per cent. That's right: zero. You read it right. Men's workload increases by nought, zilch, nix, zip, nada and diddly-squat. To put that into perspective, out of the 7,000 nappies a child will require before it's toilet trained, there's a good chance that the mother will be changing over 6,900 of them, if not all. I know of one father who hasn't changed a single nappy and the baby is seven months old. And before you answer, 'Yes, but the man's probably at work all day,' I'm no expert, but I believe children also excrete outside of business hours.

Referring to a report by the Australian Federal Office of the Status of Women called 'Juggling Time: How Australian Families Use Time', Maushart says that men who become fathers are 'even less available to participate in household tasks than before. Instead, he will work longer hours for pay – an average of 58 per cent longer during his children's pre-school years.' It is unclear if the men are working longer hours to bring home a bigger pay cheque or if they are simply doing so to escape.

There is some evidence to suggest that it may be the latter. In his book *Fat, Forty and Fired*, ex-ad man Nigel Marsh confessed that he did just this. Before he was forty and fired (I can only assume he was still fat at the time), he would sit in his car outside the house after work trying to avoid the evening chaos of getting his four children fed, bathed and in bed. Never mind about his poor wife inside who was dealing with the chaos on her own, and had been all day.

It would be comforting to think that the gross inequality in domestic and childcare work is simply and reasonably explained by the fact that the woman is at home all day and the man is at work. But I'm sorry to tell you, girls, that even in cases where the roles are reversed and men are the primary carers, women still do most of the cooking and cleaning and look after the kids at night and at the weekend. It seems that many stay-at-home dads clock off as soon as mummy walks in the door. I suspect that most stay-at-home mothers will tell you they haven't clocked off since they gave birth.

Is there no way out of this bind? I finally discover another study that gives me a small sliver of hope. Published in the *Journal of Sociology*, an article by Lyn Craig found that men's contribution to domestic work has become slightly more equal to that of women over the past 50 years. Hooray! There is hope for Chris and me yet.

My joy is short-lived. It turns out that the only reason they have become more equal is because women are doing less, not because men are doing more. It's depressing to think that in spite of half a century of women fighting for equality, men still don't consider it their responsibility to pick up a vacuum cleaner or put on a load of washing. This is why having a baby seems to turn even the most liberated women into 1950s housewives. Children require constant care, so it's not possible for women to simply lower their standards and withdraw their labour, as they have done with much of the housework. If men are not going to step up and take responsibility, women have no choice but to do it themselves.

Studies have shown that single mothers actually do less domestic work than mothers with partners, over nine hours less per week, in fact. So not only are mothers cleaning up after their kids, they are also cleaning up after their husbands. Single mothers also have more leisure time and get more sleep. I don't envy my meditation friends who are choosing to go it alone, but it's nice to know that they will experience some benefits.

There's no question in my mind that when it comes to unpaid work women are getting a raw deal. Yet it amazes me that we put up with it. How is it that we can kick arse in the boardroom but allow ourselves to get walked all over at home? In fact, when men do pitch in at home their female partners seem to be grateful that they are 'helping'. Surely a man isn't 'helping' when he washes his own shirts or cooks his own dinner. It's not 'helping' when he takes care of his children. When my client tells me that he's 'babysitting' his kids at the weekend, I shake my head in dismay. You don't babysit your own children. It's called parenting!

I wonder if this situation would change if men realised that one of the best ways to get a woman's clothes off is to wash them for her. A study by Constance T. Gager and Scott T. Yabiku published in America's *Journal of Family Issues* interviewed 7,000 married couples and revealed that men who do more housework get more sex. And Barbara Pocock, director of the Centre for Work and Life at the University of South Australia, told the *Sydney Morning Herald* that resentment over housework kills libido: 'If the resentment factor was high, that's when their sex life was not great. The best sex aid a man could use was a vacuum cleaner.'

What's perhaps more alarming is how sex is used in relationships after a child is born. The three authors of *Babyproofing Your Marriage*, Stacie Cockrell, Cathy O'Neill and Julia Stone, confess that after they had kids their enthusiasm for sex dwindled to 'folding the washing' levels. Claiming that the sex lives of new parents become so bleak, they have developed a cost–benefit analysis of giving your partner a blow job. They call it the 'Five-Minute Fix'.

For five minutes of 'physical exertion', they claim, you 'buy yourself a couple of days, maybe even a week' of peace and your partner may even 'change the next smelly nappy without being asked'. When you've spent your day cleaning up bodily fluids, what difference does a little extra make? If these authors are to be believed, motherhood really does spell the end of spontaneous, passionate and romantic romps and instead we are left with marriage-maintenance blow jobs.

A friend who has recently become a mum confides that she now only has sex when she feels obliged. Her husband is about to go on a business trip to Thailand and she says, 'He's probably going to get a massage with a happy ending, but I don't even care any more. At least I don't have to do it.'

I share my concerns with Emma. 'If our sex life is reduced to five-minute fixes,' I say, 'will Chris be reduced to a porn addict with callused hands?'

'Kase,' she replies, 'most men already are – and it has nothing to do with having children.'

When I read about the link between becoming a father and becoming a stinking-cheating-bastard-arsehole, I can see another reason why some women may come to rely on the five-minute fix. According to the book *Making Marriage Work for Dummies*, extramarital affairs are common after the birth of the first child. I think we can safely assume that it's probably not the sleep-deprived new mother that's doing the cheating. Depending on whose figures you believe, between 25 and 60 per cent of men will cheat during their marriages. Therefore, there must be a lot of husbands who are getting their five-minutes fixes and more elsewhere.

It's not just the lack of sex, however, that make men 'outsource'. It's also about lack of attention. For the first time in the relationship, the man isn't the centre of his partner's world. It makes me think about how first children get jealous and act up when the new baby arrives. I hadn't realised that husbands act up too. I wonder if it's like having two two year olds in the house. *Making Marriage Work for Dummies* outlines one scenario of how an affair happens: the man goes to work and starts noticing the younger, non-sleep-deprived woman with her pre-baby body. It starts off as a friendly chat, the husband telling his pretty colleague that his wife doesn't care about his needs any more. She'll no longer have sex with him, she's not interested in his day any more and all she wants him for is the money he brings home. The pretty young thing's heart bleeds for the poor, lonely, neglected and misunderstood man. She wants to ease his pain, so she unbuttons his fly and gives him a blow job. I embellished this story a bit, but you get the idea.

I can see how easily this can happen, and upon reflection, I think a male colleague might have even tried it on me. I must be a heartless bitch, because I ended up siding with his wife and not once did I feel compelled to offer myself to medicate his pain. Another colleague once told me that after his baby arrived he'd been demoted from head of the household to the bottom of the pecking order; he was even below the dog and the goldfish. He worked long hours and often took his business to strip clubs after work. No wonder his wife didn't feel like sex. The poor woman was practically raising the child on her own and would have been exhausted and pissed off.

I'm not saying that all men are like this. In fact, I'd like to think that even the best-case scenario of 25 per cent of men cheating is an exaggeration. But you do have to wonder if men would feel so neglected if they spent more time caring for their children. Wouldn't this make a man feel that his child is more of a joint project than a source of competition for the mother's attention?

After reading all these studies, I'm starting to wonder if feminism actually happened or if I'm just confusing it with a childhood fairy tale. Flicking through the pages of a parenting magazine later that day, I come across yet another example of how we seem to have forgotten about the revolution. I read a tip on how to save money sent in by a reader: 'Since being at home with my son, I have started making a packed lunch for my husband. This saves £25 to £40 each week, plus it helps my husband to eat healthier meals. Some days I also slip in a note saying how much I love him.'

Can you believe it? The mother is most likely up all night attending the child, probably while the husband sleeps through, yet she considers it her job to get up in the morning to make her husband's lunch. If Chris ever expects that of me, I'm quite sure the note I slip into his lunch box will not be saying 'I love you.'

I share my shock and dismay with a colleague who has just had a baby and am even more shocked and dismayed by her response. She says, 'Well, of course. Men aren't capable of caring for children the way we are. It's just not in their nature. I wouldn't trust a man to look after my baby.' I can scarcely believe what I'm hearing. Has everyone started popping Stupid Pills and no one's let me in on their stash? Just so there's no mistake, let's repeat that doozie: men are incapable of childcare.

If this were true, it would mean that the male human, despite all his evolutionary advantages, is actually less advanced than your average king penguin. The male penguin shares responsibility for looking after the egg with the mother, often incubating the egg for days on end by balancing it on its feet while the mother goes off to hunt for fish. My colleague's baby is a little boy, so I can't help but wonder if she is raising him to be as domestically useless as his father and thereby creating a rod for another woman's back in about 30 years' time.

At this rate, we'd all be better off shacking up with a sub-Antarctic bird.

# 9

# YOU CAN'T PUT IT ON YOUR CV

Having dinner with our friends Brad and Simone, Chris observes that Simone isn't drinking her wine. I haven't noticed, because throughout the evening the glass of wine in front of her is being emptied and refilled at the same rate as the rest of the table. Chris also observes that Simone seems completely sober and Brad's jokes are deteriorating rapidly.

'Somebody's got a secret,' I say mischievously.

Brad looks at Simone with a mix of love, pride and excitement, and their secret is no longer. 'I'm going to be a dad,' he bursts out.

'It's early days,' Simone says cautiously. 'We're not telling people for another six weeks.'

'Yes, but it's just Chris and Kasey.' Brad says it in such a way that makes me suspect he's also told just his best mate, just his colleagues, just his football team, just his dentist.

After the toasts and backslapping, I direct the conversation to their plans for childcare and domestic work. Simone will take a year off from her job as an office manager and Brad will continue working as an IT consultant. When I ask Brad if he's prepared for all the sleepless nights ahead, he says, matter-of-factly, 'I won't be getting up in the night because I'll have to go to work the next day.'

I bite my tongue, but what I want to say is, 'And what do you think Simone will be doing all day?'

I don't want to beat up on Brad. He's a good guy. But implicit in his view is that not only is his work more important, but what Simone will be doing all day – raising his child – isn't even considered to be work.

Most mothers I've spoken to tell me that they've never worked so hard in their lives. Jean Hampton famously wrote a letter to *The Observer* saying, 'During the thirty-five years of my working life I have worked part-time, half-time, and full-time, but when my three children were small, I worked all-the-bloody-time.'

It makes me think about my friend Sophie, who sent the email about her experiences of motherhood. It seems that the hardest part about all the unpaid, monotonous, relentless work she does in caring for the children and her husband and running the house is that it's never recognised. The 55 hours and 48 minutes of domestic work she does each week is only noticed if it doesn't get done.

But I must confess that I've been guilty of thinking like Brad too. When I started working part-time, I noticed for the first time all the mothers walking the streets with prams, sitting in parks and sipping coffee in cafes during the day. I remember thinking that they had it made. They socialised all day while their husbands went to work and earned the money.

That was before I started talking to mothers and trawling through the research on motherhood. That was before I discovered that mothers are among the most isolated groups in our society and their self-esteem has been battered by the views of people like me who assumed they spend all day lunching. I hadn't realised that those mothers I was judging were guzzling coffee because they hadn't slept for more than two hours in a row for five or six months, and that I was probably observing the only adult conversation they'd had all day, or possibly all week.

After their coffee catch-up, they all go back to their homes and have nobody to talk to until their partners come home. And if their partner is late home, they'll probably be too exhausted to engage in meaningful conversation anyway. These women have transitioned from a world where they were able to clock off at work and have the freedom to do something else to a world where they are on duty every minute of every day, of every week, of every month. There are no lunch breaks, no home times, no weekends, no holidays, no sick days. And yet we believe that daddy needs his sleep more than mummy because he has to get up the next day and do something hard, something important.

I can't even imagine what it would be like to work so hard and so relentlessly at something and not be recognised for it. If I ever have to pull an all-nighter or work at the weekend, I make sure everybody knows about it. I expect to be praised for my sacrifice and dedication. I'm sure it's a character flaw, but I thrive on social recognition. It's really important to me that my boss recognises when I've done a good job at work or when a client acknowledges that I've helped them. On the occasions when I've written articles for newspapers, I'm thrilled when people post a comment or send me an email. Even if they hate what I have said in the article or accuse me of being a 'snobby bitch' or a 'raving feminist who can't cope with the lack of male attention', I love the fact that I have made an impact and that my work has been recognised. If I become a mum, it seems I'll get none of that feedback.

Reading the parenting magazines doesn't help. I read an article in which a mother of two toddlers bravely admits that she's sick of motherhood. She says that the hard work of raising children is rarely acknowledged outside mothers' groups, and she's dispirited that her work is invisible and goes unthanked by people who should know better. 'Where's my encouragement and support during this difficult time?' she writes. 'To put it in paid-employment terms, where's my performance review? Where's my annual bonus?'

We are all complicit in perpetuating the belief that real work, the sort that you can put on your CV and talk about at dinner parties, happens outside the home. Mothering and domestic work is the engine room that enables the real world to function. Without the constant humming of this invisible engine, civilisation as we know it would break down. Politics, the economy and industry could not function if children were not mothered, mouths were not fed and houses and clothes were not cleaned. It is truly scandalous that this vital work is totally taken for granted. Yet nobody seems scandalised.

Mothering is so devalued that in many cases mothers and children are even regarded as public nuisances. We've all heard stories of women who are asked to leave restaurants because they are breastfeeding, or read letters in the newspaper from people complaining about having their Sunday brunch interrupted by children in cafes. One mum tells me that every time she has her pram out in public she feels like people are looking at her as if she's a nuisance. When I look surprised, she says, 'Can you imagine trying to catch a bus or a train in peak hour with a pram?'

There is a whole lot of whingeing going on here, isn't there? And part of me thinks that if it's all so terrible then why have children at all? In this age of education and reliable contraception, presumably all these mothers chose motherhood freely. So what are they complaining about? Should we have sympathy for these women when this is what they chose? As somebody who may well be infertile, it has crossed my mind more than once that perhaps these mothers should suck it up and be grateful that they even have kids.

From what I can tell, a lot of mothers feel this way too. They do feel lucky to have kids and they love their kids dearly, so they don't feel entitled to complain about their situations. In fact, they feel guilty about their discontentment. Because they love their children, they feel like they should love motherhood.

But it's only just occurred to me that they are not the same thing. Who in their right mind would rejoice at losing their autonomy and social status? What sane person would delight in spending every day cleaning up vomit, drool, poo and mushy food? Sleep deprivation is used as a form of torture because it erodes prisoners' confidence and mental health. Why would we assume its effects would be different on mothers simply because they are grateful to have children? I think it's reasonable to assume that most people love their children, but it's hard for me to believe that anybody could love the lifestyle that motherhood imposes on them.

Researcher Mary Boulton wrote in *On Being a Mother: A Study of Women with Pre-school Children* that, 'Although [mothers] loved their pre-school children passionately, most did not really "enjoy" life with them.' Even though women believe that mothering their children is meaningful and important, it seems that many of them would rather be doing something else. Susan Maushart points out in *The Mask of Motherhood* that motherhood is not a 'phase' or an 'opportunity': it's a way of life. 'It just so happens that it is a way of life utterly subversive to contemporary values stressing achievement, control and autonomy as the highest of adult aspirations.'

Psychologists say that when you mix together a whole lot of hard work with a big pinch of guilt, and leave out the sweetener of social recognition, you end up with the perfect recipe for postnatal depression (PND). Psychologist Paula Nicolson writes in her book *Postnatal Depression: Facing the Paradox of Loss, Happiness and Motherhood* that:

> Typical images of motherhood revolve around it being a major source of women's self-expression and satisfactions; rarely do women picture themselves, in advance, as selflessly giving, ignoring their own needs and desires and experiencing loneliness and isolation. To subscribe to this dominant myth means that the early days and months of motherhood have a double impact. The inevitable stress, exhaustion and the burden of childcare are set against each woman's fear that she is somehow 'doing it wrong'. Her experience does not relate to her dream.

Women are more likely to suffer from depression or be diagnosed with mental illness when they have young children than during any other time in their lives. Some studies reveal that 50 per cent of mothers with young children experience symptoms of intense emotional distress on a regular or continual basis. Other studies claim that it's as high as eight in ten women who experience depression or despair after becoming mothers. And, according to the research, things don't improve when the kids get older either. An article by Ranae J. Evenson and Robin W. Simon in the *Journal of Health and Social Behaviour* concludes that 'the emotional demands of parenthood at this stage of the life course may simply outweigh the emotional rewards of having children'.

It's not uncommon for women to fantasise about killing or harming their babies. Doctor and mother Penny Adams confesses having such 'black thoughts' in her book *Motherguilt*, co-authored by Ita Buttrose. She fantasised about throwing her first child out of the window or drowning her children in the bath. She had no intention of actually doing it, but these thoughts alone terrified her.

PND terrifies me. I view my depression a bit like a physical injury. If you've ever had a back injury or another kind of physical injury, you know that it will always be your weak spot. The injury never quite heals properly, and if you're not careful, or sometimes even if you are careful, it can flare up and cripple you for days or even weeks. Depression is my back injury. I sustained the 'injury' after my mother tried to commit suicide in my apartment after my father left her for another woman. It took almost two years of treatment before I recovered, but even now, from time to time, I find myself walking with an emotional limp.

When I've had serious bouts of depression in the past, I haven't been able to get out of bed or off the couch for days, sometimes even weeks. It would take me all day to muster the motivation and energy to have a shower. Some days I couldn't even do that. Cooking or shopping was beyond me, so, before Chris moved in with me, I'd only eat the things in my fridge or cupboard that didn't require preparation. Mostly this was gin and ice cream. I stopped taking Toffee for walks, and I wouldn't allow myself to go out onto my balcony because I was afraid I might jump off.

It was bad enough when it was just me that I was neglecting. What will happen if I have a child? How could I possibly take care of a child when at times I can't even take care of myself? I'm guessing that a diet of gin and ice cream is not recommended for infants.

Chris knows about my fear of PND even before I mention it. When I find a brochure about it wedged in a pile of his books, I realise that it's his fear too. I don't so much fear PND because of its effect on me; I fear it for its effects on my baby. I don't want to be a depressed mother. I don't want to actually throw my baby out a window. One night I raise my fears with Chris. 'What if I get PND?' I say.

'Then we'll deal with it,' he says calmly and confidently.

'Aren't you worried that I'll throw your baby out the window?' I push. 'It's not just about me any more; it's also about what I might do to your child.'

Chris says he's not worried, and I almost believe him. He says that as long as I tell him what I'm thinking and feeling, no matter what it is, then we'll be able to work through it together. He also tells me that it seems perfectly reasonable for a woman to go through emotional upheaval when she becomes a mother. 'If you lose your sense of identity, your independence, your income and your position in society, why wouldn't you grieve for it?' Chris says.

Freud argues that people need to express their grief in order to heal. Grief is like a bridge that takes you from your state of loss to a new state of acceptance. But the problem is, unlike other types of loss, it is not socially acceptable for a woman to grieve when she becomes a mother. She shouldn't grieve because she should be happy (which she probably is), she should be grateful (which she probably is too) and she should selflessly just get on with it (which she probably does).

In a way, it's comforting to think that if I were to become a mother then grief, and most likely depression, are inevitable simply because they are normal responses and not because I am perverse in some way. But this doesn't make it any less scary.

# 10

# WHAT IF I SUCK AT IT?

I don't just fear that I'll be a bad mother during the times when I'm depressed. What if I'm rubbish at motherhood all the time?

When I arrive home from work to discover Toffee chomping on her bone on the couch, I realise that my parenting skills leave something to be desired. Toffee knows she's not allowed to bring her bone inside. The bone has clearly spent the best part of the day in the sun. It is a disgusting hunk of fly-infested rotting flesh. The foul meat is mixing with her doggy drool and seeping into the couch. Toffee sees me and immediately rolls into the submissive position, wagging her tail and giving me her best 'aren't-I-the-cutest-puppy-in-the-world?' expression. My anger and frustration disappear instantly and my heart melts. What a gorgeous puppy dog.

I remind myself that I'm supposed to be angry, so I do my best imitation of stern. In my deepest, most assertive voice, I instruct her to get off the couch and remind her that she's not allowed to eat bones inside. I confiscate her bone and am about to put it in the bin when I see her sitting next to my foot. She's looking up at me with her big puppy-dog eyes, just as she did on the day she seduced me into buying her in the pet shop. I capitulate and give her the bone back but stipulate that she has to eat it outside.

As Toffee is happily munching on her bone outside, it occurs to me that the little bugger has just manipulated me. Again. This pattern has been going on for 12 years. Toffee jumps on everyone who comes to the door, despite 12 years of 'training'. She barks when the phone rings, despite 12 years of 'stern' remonstrations. And she picks fights with other dogs twice her size in the park, despite 12 years of my – and the larger dogs' – 'advice' to reconsider her position. She knows all these things but chooses not to obey. I may as well come out and admit it: I have raised a delinquent dog – she has no boundaries, no discipline and no respect for authority.

Surely I have failed at the first test of motherhood. If my dog-rearing skills are anything to go by, my child is sure to be stealing cars before he or she is tall enough to touch the pedals. I tell Chris of my fears as soon as he comes home from work, and he says, 'Don't worry about it, I've always raised very well-behaved cats.'

Despite Chris's assurances that I am maternal, I'm not convinced. I didn't even play with dolls as a child. I wanted dolls so I could be like everyone else. I even wanted a Cabbage Patch Kid and have never recovered from the social ostracism that resulted from not having one. My parents wouldn't let me have one, and I suspect that made me want one even more. But even if my parents had given in to my begging and pleading and claims that my life would be over if I didn't have my very own Cabbage Patch Kid, I wouldn't have known what to do with it. I never saw the point of dressing and undressing a doll, and as for pretending to feed it, what would be the point of that? It's made of plastic and fabric; it has no digestive system.

But what if my desire to have a baby is just a grown-up version of my Cabbage Patch Kid experience? What if I decide I want one because everyone else has one – or, worse, because I've been told that I might not be able to have one? And if I do eventually get my real-life Cabbage Patch Kid, will I know what to do with it? Will I be able to cope with it?

I'm a little reassured to discover the counter-argument to the 'motherhood-is-in-your-genetic-code' theory in the pages of many of the books on motherhood. Many scientists and clinicians believe that mothering is a skill, just like any other, that you have to learn. Giving birth does not trigger an automatic download of the mothering software into your brain. Apparently it has always been this way. Because we no longer live in tribes and haven't been involved in mothering other children of the group, we come to parenthood uninitiated and ignorant. We are tripped up by the expectation that mothering is innate. So when we discover at 2 a.m. that we have no idea how to soothe our screaming babies, our worry, exhaustion and frustration is also compounded by a sense of inadequacy and failure.

This is reassuring to me. If motherhood is learned, then I should have no problem. I've always been a good student and have aced tests (with the exception of maths and woodwork). But on the other hand, there would be few people who are more uninitiated and ignorant in the ways of mothering than I am. I've never even been alone with a child before. Nappy technology perplexes me. I noticed in the supermarket the other day that nappy manufacturers go to great lengths to explain about the super-absorbency layers and contoured sides, but none of them include instructions for how to put the damn things on. How is a new parent supposed to know what to do? They look like origami.

With no in-built mothering skills and no previous exposure to mothering in which to learn these skills, I have no way of knowing if I have the aptitude to mother. I don't like doing things I'm not good at.

I imagine that in many ways motherhood is even harder now than it was for our grandmothers' generation. Sure, their husbands did even less than husbands today, but at least they didn't have to deal with the disappointment of expecting otherwise. The standards of motherhood and pressures of intensive mothering have also changed. When a baby cried, our grandmothers didn't feel compelled to settle it immediately or else risk an increase in cortisol, which will shrink the baby's hippocampus, which will cause anxiety and attachment issues later in life, which will turn them into a sociopath and result in an exposé in a newspaper titled 'The Mother Who Created a Monster'. Crying used to be considered good for the baby's lungs, and if the noise got too much for the mother she could just shut the baby in the cupboard for a while and enjoy a quiet, guilt-free cup of tea. She also would have most likely had her mother, mother-in-law, sisters and aunts living in the same neighbourhood and able to help out. And let's face it, beating a child with a wooden spoon would surely have faster results than the naughty seat or threatening to confiscate their Xbox.

My fears about motherhood are exacerbated as I watch a news report about people who bought miniature pigs as pets only to discover that they weren't miniature at all. The pigs have transformed from cute, pink, little cuddly things into enormous, dirty, smelly standard pigs: a bit like teenagers. It occurs to me that when I am imagining myself as a mother my mental image is of me looking hot (the weight loss is from breastfeeding), holding a gorgeous little baby who is staring up at me gooing and gaaing as if I am the only person in the world. My mental picture hasn't yet extended to a moody teenager who only speaks to me when they want money or to tell me to fuck off when I ask them what time they will be home.

I have hardly even thought about a defiant toddler who will punish me with a temper tantrum in the supermarket for not buying lollies. My mum still has the note I wrote to her when I was five. It said: 'I hat mum' (I've never been very good at spelling). In my mind, my darling little baby doesn't have the fine motor skills to hold a pencil, let alone the strength of will to tell me they hate me.

When people say, 'Enjoy them when they're young, they grow up so quickly,' are they actually saying that we should make the most of it when they are babies because things go downhill rapidly after that? It's a shame the guide-dog programme can't be extended to babies – you know, when you get to look after and play with gorgeous little puppies for a year and then hand them over to somebody else to train.

I wish there was some way of knowing definitively and ahead of time if I will be good at mothering and if I'll enjoy it. The authors of *Do I Want to Be a Mom?* claim that 'You can't always predict whether you have the strength to survive them with your sanity intact.' They quote a woman named Sandy who says, 'It took so much energy. I just didn't have it. I tried, but I just didn't have it. I don't know how other women do it. It'll be a long time before my kids understand, and I don't know if they will ever forgive me, but I hope someday they do.'

When I consider all the women I know who have babies, some of them love motherhood and have embraced it as if they have been doing it all their lives, but other friends haven't. What scares me is that I've been unable to predict who will take to motherhood and who won't. I am surprised when a friend who I would have thought was born to be a mother claims she doesn't like it at all. She has never been particularly ambitious in a professional sense, so it isn't like she is regretting giving up her career. In fact, she's never really had a job or a career that has been particularly satisfying. I ask her what she would prefer to be doing if she wasn't a mother. She replies, 'I don't know what I want to do, but I know it's not this.' And then I've seen über-ambitious colleagues who swear they will be back at work three months after their baby is born completely embrace motherhood and not come back to work at all.

Research shows that the more highly educated and established in your career you are, the harder you're going to find motherhood. I suppose that when you have become accustomed to being autonomous and in control, the more your life has to change when you become a mother.

I search through books and scientific journals to see if I can find predictive criteria to determine mothering potential and satisfaction. I find a study that predicts marital happiness, but there is nothing on maternal happiness. I ask my psychologist if he knows of any studies, but he doesn't. He says that good mothers need to have self-insight and empathy, but he doesn't know of any definitive predictive criteria. But he assures me that with all of his years of experience he can predict it with a 'clinical feel', and he is quite sure that not only will I be good at motherhood, I'll also enjoy it.

This is nice to hear, but my friend Paul, who most certainly has empathy and self-insight, once told me that if he had his time over he wouldn't have kids – not because he didn't love them, but because he loves them too much. He says that he'd never experienced such intense emotion before having kids. It breaks his heart when his daughter gets teased at school or when his twelve-year-old son is devastated because he's the only one in his group who doesn't have a girlfriend. 'It hurts to love someone so much,' he once told me. 'I can handle my own ups and downs, but it guts me to experience theirs.'

Once I scratch beneath the surface of the 'perfect-mother veneer' that so many women feel they must construct, it is truly startling how many mothers will admit they preferred their life without children or at the very least are ambivalent about motherhood. Even complete strangers tell me they regret motherhood, as if they are trying to prevent me from catching an incurable disease.

As I sit in a cafe reading the book *Childfree and Loving It!* by Nicki Defago, a tired- and frazzled-looking woman at the table next to mine leans over and says, 'Don't do it, don't believe what they tell you, it's not worth it.' When she fell pregnant in her late 30s, she felt like the lucky one amongst all of the other women she knew who were unsuccessfully trying to conceive. 'But now I think that they are the lucky ones,' she says. 'They escaped the life sentence of hard labour.'

Reading Nicki Defago's book further, there are heartbreaking and terrifying anecdotes aplenty to scare the shit out of those considering motherhood. One woman says, 'I became a parent reluctantly, and always knew I'd made the wrong decision. My child is now a fine and loving adult, and does not know that secretly I still terribly regret letting myself think I ought to go along with the prevailing customs. I would have been a far happier person as a non-parent.' Another confesses, 'If I had known how having children would make me feel, I wouldn't have had them, so presumably my earlier reservations were somewhat justified . . . The biological "rub" is that you can never truly know in advance how you will respond to this mammoth event. If we did, not many of us would reproduce.'

This one scares me the most:

> I hate being a parent. I hate being Mommy. My kids are okay people, even cute sometimes, but I don't feel any great love for them. I take good care of them, I'd do everything I could to help them and protect them, but if I had a chance to go back in time, I would not have these children. You're probably expecting some horror story. There isn't one, other than that every day of my life, I wish I didn't have children . . . I hate the pressures and expenses of parenthood. The rewards seem so few, and not long lasting . . . I feel like I'm not my own person any more. Even my husband thinks I'm Mommy, not his wife . . . It's like being in a job you dislike, a job that bores you, that sucks your soul out, except you can't leave this job and go home. It's always there waiting for you, needing to be done. This is not the kind of thing people like to talk about or admit to themselves or anyone else . . . [I am] counting the days until the kids leave home and life seems worthwhile again. I guess this is what happens when people have kids without really thinking about whether they truly want to become parents.

Mothering is so permanent. In my privileged life with so many options and opportunities, it is the only thing I can think of that I can't undo. If I don't like my job I can quit it and get a new one, sell my apartment and buy or rent somewhere else, move countries, lose weight (if my desire to get back into my skinny jeans ever outweighs my desire for Cadbury Creme Eggs), change my hair colour, break up with Chris and find a new boyfriend, and change my social circle. But once I am a mother, I will always be a mother. There is no exchange receipt, and the job is a job for life.

More than ever, I now know that parenting doesn't end when the kids leave home. When my dad left my mother, I was living happily and independently in Holland. I was a grown-up; I had my own life. Yet the fallout from both their actions truly devastated me. My father, presumably thinking that his fathering job was done, essentially walked away from our family and started a new life with his new wife. And given that his children are now in their 30s, it would seem reasonable to assume that as a father he is no longer required. But that was before I had experienced it myself.

Now I know differently. Even now, years later, and potentially on the verge of starting my own family, I am acutely aware of how much power my father still has in my life. When my father comes to town and 'doesn't have time' to see me, the rejection feels like a blade through the heart. It takes days, if not weeks, to stop the bleeding. No matter how hard I try to approach the situation as a grown-up, deep down I will always be the little girl whose daddy doesn't want her any more. I have become another one of those women with 'father issues', and it doesn't seem possible to outrun them. So I am quite sure that once I become a parent, I will always be a parent, and whether I like it or not, I'll always have the power to break my child's heart.

Chris isn't concerned so much about whether or not we'll like having a baby; he's more concerned about whether or not the baby will like having us. Chris is not your typical blokey man. He's into literature, art and music and probably couldn't even identify the football teams, let alone name the players. And as for me, well, I've never been able to master the skill of catching a ball. 'What if we have a really masculine child who is into sport and monster-truck racing?' Chris says. 'He won't be able to relate to me.'

We agree that if the worst were to happen and we did end up with an athletic child, we could outsource the football to Emma. She goes to the football regularly, so she could take junior along. And Jules used to be the captain of the Western Australian women's cricket team, so she could be in charge of teaching ball skills. But as for the monster-truck racing: we're screwed.

'I just hope we have a girl or a gay boy,' Chris says.

When I relay Chris's concerns to Jules, she laughs and says he's got to be the only man alive who is hoping that his child will be a poofter.

# 11

# THE BABY SWITCH

'I'm not a violent person,' my friend Danielle tells me, taking a sip of her cabernet, 'but I just want to kill them.'

I surreptitiously look round the cafe at the nearby tables, just in case anyone overheard her telling me how she feels about women who wish they'd never had children, or who speak disparagingly about their children.

Danielle is a 40-something account manager in the IT industry. She's vivacious, optimistic and one of the most open and generous people I know. I've never known her to utter a word in anger – until, that is, I bring up the topic of people who say that they wish they'd never had kids.

Also in Danielle's sights are people who have accidental pregnancies. 'Why are they having unprotected sex if they don't want a baby? They know the risks. It's like jumping off a cliff and being surprised when you hit the bottom. I just think, "You fucking cow, just have the baby and give it to me."'

After years of unsuccessful fertility treatment, she is having to accept that she will never be a mother. She started IVF when she was in her late 30s because she and her partner Mark had a chemical incompatibility and were unable to conceive naturally. Initially she convinced herself that if she was fertile enough, it wouldn't matter about the incompatibility of Mark's sperm. But it did matter. When

Danielle decided to stop IVF, she felt like a complete failure and dreaded having to face a lifetime of 'So, do you have kids?'

'It hurts every time people ask,' she says. 'Especially when people say "I'm so sorry", it's like dealing with a death. I constantly have to admit that I can't have kids, that I failed. It never stops hurting.

'Having children is so easy for most people,' Danielle says. 'One of my best friends was complaining that she gets pregnant at the drop of a hat. People don't realise what they are saying. It's like if you've just lost somebody in a car accident, and somebody says, "I hope you crash your car and die." But then with people who are sensitive and reserved about discussing pregnancy it's almost as bad. In fact, facing the pity can even be worse.'

Danielle looked into the options of using donor sperm, but Mark made it quite clear that it wasn't an option. He never articulated why. He was so adamant about it that his reasons weren't even discussed. He felt the same about adoption. Consequently, Danielle spent more time than she probably should have contemplating having a one-night stand.

'I spent a lot of time wondering how you get somebody to not wear a condom. But at my age I know it would take more than one night. And when the kid asks about who their dad is, I'd have to say, "I don't know, I just slept around for a while until I got pregnant,"' she says. She also thought about going through IVF as a single woman and not telling Mark. If she conceived with the donor sperm, she'd just let him believe they conceived naturally. But she didn't go through with either deception because she couldn't bring herself to hurt Mark. 'I realised that my relationship with him is more important than having kids,' she says.

From what she tells me, dealing with childlessness sounds a lot like grieving for a loved one. Initially you battle to get through every minute, then it's every hour, then every day and then every week. It's only after you've grieved sufficiently that you can start moving on. You keep grieving until one day the balance changes and you realise that you've got more life than grief.

'I actively worked to turn my mind around,' Danielle says. 'I went from being resentful of every fertile woman on the planet to being happy for them.' She's thrown herself back into her life, cultivated some hobbies, goes out to dinner more and has learned that it's OK to go to the zoo or watch *Ice Age* without kids. But she still looks longingly at every pregnant woman and wishes she could go through that.

I ask Danielle what made her stop the IVF cycles and she said, 'I didn't want to be suicidal any more because I was afraid that one day I might actually do it.' Each IVF cycle took Danielle through altitude sickness-inducing highs to bottomless lows, and even worse than the disappointment of not getting a baby at the end of each failed IVF cycle was knowing she'd have to go through it all again. She also wanted her old life back. 'I was so tired of the needles and people sticking things up me,' she says. 'I realised that I needed to live the life I had rather than the one I wanted. I was ruining the life I had by trying to get the one I wanted.'

Mark didn't cope with IVF very well either. 'He retreated into his work and stopped looking after himself,' Danielle says. 'And I was so self-obsessed. I spent so much energy just trying to stay alive.'

It's not surprising that Danielle and Mark's relationship was damaged by the IVF experience. It took them a while to reconnect as friends and then as lovers. 'It took a couple of years to start enjoying sex again,' Danielle says. 'There was so much pressure on what is meant to be fun and intimate. We eventually went back to being lovers rather than two people trying to make a baby.'

Danielle assures me that childlessness hurts less over time and that she has moved on . . . mostly. Despite having 'moved on', her age and her history of infertility, Danielle still hopes that one day it'll 'just happen' naturally. Talking to Danielle breaks my heart but I think this residual hope is the most upsetting part of all. Danielle has as much chance of conceiving a baby naturally as she does of a stork delivering one to her door, yet she still lives in hope. What will happen to Danielle when she hits the menopause and she can no longer cling to the hope that it will 'just happen'?

As soon as I say goodbye to Danielle, I start to cry. Her story is so heartbreaking; how could I not cry for her? I wonder if Danielle is crying too. Does she still cry when nobody is looking?

Later that day I phone Emma to tell her about my conversation with Danielle. 'I don't want to be like that,' I say. 'I couldn't bear the grief.' Despite Danielle's optimistic and cheery disposition, there is an unmistakable sadness lying just below the surface. It's like a wound that will never heal, one that will go on festering every time somebody asks if she has children, and every Mother's Day, and every time she feels excluded from family functions, and every time she sees a pregnant woman.

I tell Emma that Danielle didn't always want children. She sailed through her 20s and early 30s with ambivalence and the confidence that she could worry about it later. She used to be just like Emma and me, until the baby switch flickered to life and all of a sudden she wanted a baby with every fibre of her being. But when her switch was glowing red, she was already an old lady in fertility years. Mark's incompatible sperm didn't help the situation, but even if he had been producing Olympic swimmers, Danielle's eggs were already in the hydrotherapy pool doing old-lady water aerobics.

Emma's first encounter with the baby switch was with her friend Nicola. Nicola was an events manager, and not only did she organise parties, she also attended them. She was known as 'Nicola the Party Girl'. Emma saw her at a function a couple of years ago where she grabbed Emma's arm and said, 'Oh my God, I want a baby.' She would have been the last person in the room Emma would have picked as wanting a baby. But all of a sudden Nicola could talk or think of nothing else. Within a year, Nicola had quit the industry, married and had a baby. Nicola was one of the lucky ones. Her switch had come on when she was young enough to do something about it.

'The switch scares the hell out of me,' Emma says. 'What if it flicks on when it's too late? I don't want to be fucked up by grief when I'm older.'

Emma and I conclude that having a baby is a gamble. We'd be gambling that we'd like it and gambling against the possibility of the switch flicking on when it's too late. This thought stays with me all day and into the evening. I can't stop thinking of Danielle's sadness and the void she seems unable to fill. As I climb into bed and snuggle up next to Chris, I feel a faint, yet undeniable, power surge to my baby switch.

And no, that's not a sexual metaphor. Get your mind out of the gutter.

# 12

# BAD BUSINESS CASE

In the days following my conversation with Danielle, I can't shake the thought of desperately wanting a baby and not being able to have one. But neither can I face the prospect of having a baby only to discover I've made a terrible – and irreversible – mistake. The problem I have is that, as heartbreaking as Danielle's story is, the management consultant in me has been trained to examine all the evidence, weighing up what people tell me against the statistics and data.

To break the impasse and come to a decision, I decide to do what any self-respecting management consultant would do in my position: I'll crunch the numbers, develop a business case and see how parenting stacks up in a cost–benefit analysis.

Based on all the data and most of the anecdotal evidence, things are not looking good for parenthood. The studies don't lie: having children is bad for your marriage and sex life, terrible for your finances, diabolical for your identity, your career and your waistline, and should be listed in the American Psychiatric Association's *Diagnostic and Statistical Manual of Mental Disorders*.

If I were a management consultant advising a client on whether or not to make a child 'investment', I'd have to tell them to avoid it like the plague. A child would be an even worse prospect than selling pets via an online mail-order pet store.

You don't have to look far to find evidence for this conclusion. Take the results of a 2003 survey from *Good Housekeeping* magazine of 1,000 readers, for example: 90 per cent of respondents claimed that motherhood damaged their careers, 60 per cent said it damaged their relationships with family and friends, and half said it damaged their sex lives. (Based on the anecdotal evidence I've collected, I suspect the other half is lying.) The editor sums up the findings by saying, 'Our survey paints a devastating picture of a woman so drained of her resources that all her vital relationships are in danger. It helps explain exactly why the birth rate is plummeting.'

And remember, this is *Good Housekeeping* we're talking about here, a magazine whose circulation depends on its target readers thinking that motherhood is a good thing. Unlike *Esquire*, *GQ* or *Playboy*, the editor of *Good Housekeeping* has a vested interest in women being so well-disposed to parenting and all things family that the prospect of popping out a few more kids is as appealing as another recipe for casserole. I figure that if the editor of *Good Housekeeping* can't manage to put a positive spin on motherhood, then this business case is dead in the water.

And yet people do it. And then, having made one 'bad investment', as if throwing good money after bad, many people do it again, and again.

But perhaps I'm being too short-term in my thinking. What about the long horizon? How does that alter the business case? Not much, as it turns out: children are not even a good long-term investment to guard against loneliness in old age. Studies have shown that childless people are no lonelier in their later years than those with children. Let's face it, most of us are going to end up in a nursing home eventually, with only Girl Guides and people on community-service orders for company. I suppose those without children are at least spared the disappointment of expecting better treatment from their children.

Nicki Defago sums it up in *Childfree and Loving It!*: 'In a cruel twist, real loneliness hits mothers who've devoted their lives to their children with little thought for themselves . . . It's the loneliness of rejection, when your grown-up kids visit, but you know it's out of duty; they move away or they don't invite you for Christmas. Babies are sweet-smelling bundles of hope and purpose, but they only stay for a while.'

I did it myself. When I left home and moved to another city, I gave my mother 24 hours' notice. At the time I couldn't fathom why my mum was upset and cried every time I spoke to her on the phone.

So why do people do it? Why do we have children when it's such a bad deal? People say that when their child looks at them and smiles, it's all worthwhile. But can a smile adequately compensate for the magnitude of ongoing 'losses'? I could keep reading books about motherhood, trawling through science and psychology journals, and accosting every mother I encounter to ask about her experiences, but it's clear that I'm not going to find a clear and unambiguous answer from the research. Sooner or later I just have to accept that motherhood is bloody hard and it requires enormous and ongoing sacrifice. And, let's face it, gender inequality is part of the deal as well. I can only assume that if I am to become a mother, there will be days when I will be enriched by a simple smile and other days when I will long for my freedom and be pissed off and resentful that my life has changed so much more than Chris's.

After all my reading and researching, I figure it all boils down to one question: am I prepared to put my dreams and plans on hold for all those years I'd be raising a child, or perhaps even sacrifice them entirely?

What are my dreams and plans? I'm actually not sure if I have anything on my must-do-before-I-die list that I haven't done already, or couldn't do with a baby, or couldn't postpone for a couple of decades. I've climbed the corporate ladder as far as I need to go to be satisfied; all my career boxes have been ticked. I've travelled a lot. Sure, there are still places left to see, but I don't have a burning desire to see them. There is barely enough room to swing a cat in my apartment, but while it would be nice to upgrade, I wouldn't feel like I was missing out if I didn't.

A few months ago when I confided in a colleague that I'd lost my give-a-shit and was totally bored with life and work, he had said that if I'm bored with my life now when I'm in my 30s, imagine how I'm going to feel when I'm in my 50s. Then he said, 'If you have children, your life will never be boring.' While I now suspect that spending all day, every day changing nappies, puréeing food, doing laundry and singing 'The Wheels On the Bus' can indeed at times be boring, I do understand the point he was trying to make.

When Emma rings and asks, 'If you don't have kids, what will you do instead?' I don't have a ready answer. In my 20s when people asked me where I saw myself in five years' time, I could tell them in great detail. Ten years from now, when I look into my future all I see is a blank page. Is it wrong to have a baby because I can't think of anything else to do instead? Does it mean I no longer have any imagination or ambition?

I feel another power surge to my baby switch and tell myself that I feel this way not because of a lack of ambition or imagination but because it's the right time in my life to become a mother. I've done all that I need to do to complete the childless independent-woman phase of my life. And I'm bloody lucky that I discovered my fertility expiration date and that I have Chris in my life so I can do something about it.

I wonder if choosing motherhood with some knowledge of the sacrifice involved will inoculate me against the resentment about the inequality. Will it help to remind myself on the hard days that I chose motherhood with my eyes wide open because I came to the conclusion that I didn't have anything better to do with my life?

When I announce to Emma that I've decided to have a baby, she says, 'I'm not surprised. I thought you'd reach that conclusion eventually.'

When I tell Chris, he says, 'Well, let's get to it then.'

# 13

# PUT YOUR LEGS IN THE AIR LIKE YOU JUST DON'T CARE

'Let me explain it to you in terms you'll understand,' my friend Jamie begins. 'Imagine you have a giant box of chocolates and you are told that you have to eat them all. The first few are great. You enjoy them. The next few are still OK, but you've had enough now. But that doesn't matter. You have to keep eating, keep eating, keep eating. You really want to stop now and you've eaten so many you feel like chocolate is the last thing in the world you want or will ever want again. You hate that you're hating it, because chocolate has always been one of your favourite things. You worry that if you keep stuffing chocolates down your throat you may be turned off chocolate for life. But you have to keep eating, keep eating, keep eating. And then when you've finished the whole box, you are given another box and told that you have to eat that too.'

This is Jamie's attempt to explain what trying to get pregnant does to your sex life. He'd been complaining about it when he was undergoing sex under duress and, having no understanding of infertility and being completely insensitive, I'd said, 'Well, it must be fun trying. Aren't you guys always complaining that you never get enough sex from your wives?'

I now know what a stupid thing to say that was.

And that's a man's point of view. If men get sick of sex when they typically are up for it any time, anywhere and anyhow, imagine what it's like for a woman. I don't know about you, but I need certain conditions to be in the mood. I need some romance or lust (or at the very least a couple of gin and tonics). I need to be feeling sexy, as in not hormonal, not fat, not tired, not distracted. More than anything, I need sex to be about the connection between my partner and me.

Unfortunately, the rules are different when you're trying to conceive. Welcome to the world of conception sex. In this world, the idea that sex is about a deeper connection between you and your partner is a luxury that you can ill afford. Instead, sex is a means to an end, one that's entirely utilitarian and clinical. In the world of conception sex, bonking is reduced to mucus consistency, body temperature and circled dates in the diary. Sending Chris a meeting request for a shag is about as romantic as it gets.

And we're only one month in.

There are two schools of thought when it comes to conception sex. The first is the Gandhi school. The basic tenet of the Gandhi school is that less is more. Its hallmarks are restraint and control. Advocates of this approach advise 'conserving the sperm' – apparently Gandhi was celibate in his 30s to conserve his 'vital fluids' – for two or three days prior to ovulation and then have sex once every two days. This is the quality-over-quantity approach. The second school is the Tiger Woods approach. The Tiger Woods approach, by contrast, which was advised by my practitioner of Chinese medicine, advocates having sex all day, every day (although, and this is a novel departure from the pure Tiger Woods approach, it's recommended that the same two people are involved on each occasion).

I soon discover that my Chinese medicine practitioner is a sadist for advising the Tiger Woods approach. It's amazing how quickly the novelty wears off. By the fifth day, I am no longer appreciative of Chris's foreplay efforts. I don't have the heart to tell him that in this case the rule that 'a gentleman should go down before he goes up' doesn't apply, and if it's all the same to him could we just get on with it already. And it's started to affect our social life. Emma tells me that she's arranged a dinner with some friends, but she's not inviting me because I have to stay at home and have sex.

By the end of the first sexathon, I breathe a sigh of relief that I can now have a rest. But I'm also overcome with excitement and anticipation at the prospect of having made a baby. I can't quite get my head around the fact that we are trying to make a person. If we manage to conceive, in nine months' time a person will come out. It will have its own needs, dreams, personality and bad habits. It is almost inconceivable that we could be capable of producing something so complex and magnificent. The most sophisticated thing my body has made prior to this is a poo. I wonder if my body is up to the task. Let's face it, the shift from making a poo to making a baby is quite a leap.

Two weeks after ovulation, I pop out of the office to buy some lunch and something strange happens. Usually I'm a turkey-and-salad-on-multigrain-bread-with-no-butter-or-salt kind of girl. But today I can't keep my eyes off all the disgusting salty fried food. The potato cakes serenade me, the chips whisper sweet nothings to me and the fried chicken is beckoning suggestively. For the first time ever, I give in to their overtures and order two pieces of fried chicken, with chips and extra salt.

As my order is being prepared, it occurs to me that there can only be one possible explanation for my radical change of taste. I'm pregnant! I must be. What other explanation can there be? Now I think about it, aren't my boobs feeling a little warmer than usual? I look around the cafe to make sure nobody is looking at me and then sneakily cop a feel of my boobs. Yep, definitely warmer, and bigger too. There's at least a full handful on each side. I'm just about to call Chris with the news when I decide that I should do a pregnancy test first just to make sure. I quickly scoff down my fried feast and rush off to the chemist.

On my walk to the chemist, I calculate the date of my maternity leave and make a mental note to check the corporate policy about when I need to inform my company. With growing excitement, I boldly ask the shop assistant for a pregnancy test. Previously when I'd bought pregnancy tests it was always accompanied by a sense of dread and embarrassment. I was convinced the shop assistant had judged me to be a slut, and on some irrational and childish level I feared she'd phone my mum and tell on me. I'd try to make a pact with God (yes, the very same one I'm not sure I believe in) that I'd never have irresponsible sex again if he could just spare me the embarrassment of getting one of those over-zealous shop assistants who insisted on reading out loud the instructions on the back of the box.

Not this time. In fact, it wouldn't bother me if she reads the instructions so loudly that everyone in the shop hears. I don't shove the test guiltily and hurriedly into my handbag as soon as it touches the counter but instead allow it to linger there momentarily on the off chance that someone I know should happen by and see me. In fact, it's going to take all the restraint I can muster not to take a photo of the double lines on the wee-stick and post it on Facebook.

As the assistant hands over my change, she says, 'Good luck.' I used to hate it when they said this. I always assumed the assistant was wishing me luck not to be pregnant. 'Good luck' was a euphemism for 'Let's hope you've dodged the bullet and you're not another irresponsible floozy bringing an unwanted child into an overpopulated world who you'll be unable to support and will inevitably be a drain on the public purse.' This time I decide to take 'Good luck' at face value and hurry back to work to pee on the stick.

As I'm waiting for the second line to appear on the stick, I compose in my mind what I will say to Chris. Do I ring up and announce the good news that he's going to be a dad straight away or do I wait until he says, 'How are you?' so I can reply, 'Pregnant'? Or is it best to wait until tonight? I can bring home a bottle of wine and when he's about to pour me a glass, I can say, 'Not for me, thanks, it's not good for our baby.'

I look down at the stick and notice that the second line hasn't appeared yet. I double-check my watch. It's been three minutes, so it should be there. I can't decide what's faulty, the stick or my watch, so

I wait a few more minutes. Still no line. The stick must be broken. That must be why they put two sticks in the box. The manufacturer's quality control must not be very good.

I pee on the second stick, but my bladder is empty so I only manage a few drops. Will that void the test? Three minutes later and there's still no second line. Another three minutes and the line is still playing hide-and-seek. I must have done it wrongly. Perhaps I was silly to try doing this myself; I'm terrible with anything vaguely scientific. I should have called in the professionals – Jules and Brandy – just like when we did Chris's sperm test.

Maybe I need fresh wee rather than a couple of drops of the dregs. Reading the more detailed instructions on the leaflet inside the box, I discover that early-morning wee is stronger and therefore better. That must be what I'm doing wrong. I stop off at a different chemist on the way home to buy another test and feel a bit like an addict buying drugs at different stores so as not to leave a trail. I buy a different brand of test, because clearly the quality-control team employed by the first brand are incompetent.

A sleepless night and a long wait until morning. But when is morning? I mean, really, when does morning begin? The manufacturer doesn't specify. Do they mean just after midnight or when the sun comes up? And would that be sunrise in winter or summer? At 2.34 a.m. I am certain that it's morning, by any reasonable person's definition, so I creep out of bed to pee on the stick. At just after 3 a.m. I return to bed, having just buried two negative wee-sticks at the bottom of the rubbish bin. A seed of doubt has sprouted in my mind, but I trample on it. I'm pregnant. I must be pregnant. Aren't my boobs a little bit bigger than normal? Aren't I feeling hungrier? Surely I wouldn't have ingested five billion calories for a fried lunch the previous day if I weren't pregnant?

Three days and sixteen wee-sticks later, my period arrives. Not even I can delude myself that it's implantation bleeding. When I tell Chris that I'm not pregnant, he says, 'I know, puss cat. The rubbish bin is full of pregnancy tests.'

As month two comes around, our friends have plenty of advice. Chris's friend Philipa suggests I do a headstand after sex. Gravity is supposed to help the sperm swim in the direction of the egg. I look at her in disbelief. Surely the female body is engineered better than this. Philipa admits that it could quite possibly be rubbish, but says she conceived her daughter the first month she tried it. Chris and I agree that we'll add a headstand to our repertoire, thinking that we have nothing to lose.

The next day after the headstand I have a headache and I feel nauseous. For a moment, I indulge in the fantasy and delusion that I'm pregnant. But only for a moment. According to my calculations, I'm not due to ovulate for another two days, so pregnancy would be impossible right now. The headache persists for several days, so I book in to get a massage. The massage therapist tells me that my neck muscles are tight and asks me what I've been doing.

'Standing on my head,' I say sheepishly.

The therapist laughs. She's on to me. 'Would that be during or after sex?' she asks.

It's amazing how a couple of minutes can make all the difference. If I'd injured myself during sex, I would be a wild, crazy sex kitten. But since I did it after sex, I'm just an infertile, gullible loser with poor upper-body strength. The therapist suggests that instead of doing a headstand I should stick some pillows under my bum and cycle my legs in the air. As I'm lying on the bed with my legs in the air for the second time that day, I say to Chris, 'Do you remember when we used to have sex purely because it was fun and because we wanted to?'

'It'll be like that again soon,' Chris says. The eternal optimist.

I say nothing because I worry that it won't ever be like that again. What if sex is like bourbon? We all have a bourbon: the drink we binged on when we were teenagers, ended up vomiting into a gutter and vowed never to touch again. Even the smell of it makes you ill. Bourbon is my drink, the drink that I overdosed on in my teens and to which I can never go back. What if bingeing on sex has the same effect as bingeing on bourbon?

I also start to worry about Chris's ego. I've read in a number of books that men do not cope well with sex under duress. My assumption that a man is always up for a quickie is clearly wrong. Men hate the pressure of being forced to perform on command. But even worse, they can end up worrying that we love their sperm more than we love them. When Brandy asks me when was the last time I gave Chris a blow job, I can't remember. We have so much sex around the time I'm ovulating that I don't feel like it when I'm not. And when I'm ovulating, his sperm is too valuable to waste. 'Spit or swallow, hon,' Brandy said. 'You need to let him know he's more to you than just a donor.'

As month three rolls around, I make the ultimate sacrifice. I 'waste' Chris's precious sperm and give him a blow job. It does cross my mind more than once that I could perhaps spit it into a jar and then use a syringe. Waste not, want not, as they say. I also make a mental note that it takes longer than five minutes. I'll have to work on my technique if I'm going to resort to the 'five-minute fix' when I become a mother.

By the fourth month, I'm convinced we are doing it wrongly. I do some more research into fertility and conception and discover that a woman is only fertile for one to two days per month. It's time to abandon the quantity approach and try for quality instead.

Unfortunately, this shift coincides with our flight from Melbourne to London. As we're in the departure lounge, I feel like I'm ovulating. I'm not going to gross you out by describing it. Let's just say that it involves ovulation mucus and leave it at that. As soon as the plane is in the air and the seatbelt sign is switched off, I make my way to the toilets with an ovulation stick in hand. Ovulation sticks work a lot like pregnancy tests. You wee on them, and if you are ovulating then a line appears. I quite like these tests. They are ridiculously expensive, but, unlike pregnancy tests, it's very satisfying to know that at least once a month I will pass the test. I wasn't expecting to pass the test on a 24-hour flight, however.

I rush back to my seat to tell Chris that I'm ovulating and he says,

'Looks like I'm about to get lucky.'

'But Chris, my fertile window could only be 24 hours,' I explain. 'By the time we get to London we may be too late.'

Chris smiles mischievously, 'We could put in our application for the mile high club.'

I used to think joining the mile high club was so cool, but I've never had the guts to do it. Here's my big chance to earn my membership, but I don't want to. I don't want to conceive my child with a quickie in a stinky aeroplane toilet. Plane toilets are disgusting even when they're clean, and this one is already starting to smell.

I agonise over the decision for a couple of hours, the whole time imagining my precious little egg sitting in my fallopian tube like a wallflower worrying that a boy will never ask her to dance. 'We can't miss this month,' I say to Chris. 'This could be my last month of fertility; it could be our last chance.' I decide to take another look at the toilet cubicle to see if I can bring myself to do it.

It's not until I'm working out the logistics of how Chris and I could squeeze into the same toilet cubicle that I realise what an achievement membership of the mile high club really is. Not only is it a feat of exhibitionism; it's also a feat in acrobatics. How do two adults manage to fit into a cubicle without contorting their bodies in some way? I don't know about you, but I find it hard to get into the mood when my head is squashed against a toilet wall, I'm breathing through my mouth so I don't have smell the toilet stench, I'm trying to stop my clothes from falling onto the soggy, wee-covered floor and I can hear the flight attendants chatting about swine flu just outside the door. Initially I feel more relief than disappointment when I conclude that we simply can't fit into the toilet.

Halfway through the flight, I start to have second thoughts. I can't bear the thought of being childless for ever simply because I was too much of a princess to have sex in a smelly coffin-sized box with a wee-soaked floor. I suggest to Chris that we have sex during our one-hour stopover at Hong Kong airport. 'I'm up for it if you are,' Chris says. We spend the first half-hour searching the airport for an appropriate place to shag. Hong Kong airport is clearly not designed for ovulating couples with fertility issues. The only suitable place we can find is a disabled toilet with a 'Do Not Enter' sign on the door. Chris doesn't want to go in because of the sign, but I convince him that it's our only option. 'Well, let's be quick,' he snaps. I can hear the tension in his voice. We rush into the toilet when nobody is looking and quickly drop our pants.

As it turns out, Chris isn't 'up' for it. Chris looks around at the filthy toilet and says, 'This is really disgusting.'

'Don't look at it,' I say as I make a half-arsed attempt at foreplay. 'Let's just get on with it.' But the mood has become decidedly flaccid. Neither of us is in any condition to have sex.

There is a knock on the door and we hurriedly pull up our pants, straighten our clothes and leave. A man in a uniform standing outside gives us a stern look, and we hurry off to our boarding gate without looking back.

Back on the plane, Chris and I laugh about what just happened. But we both know that yet another month has just ticked by.

# 14

## YES, YOU ARE OLD, AND NO, YOU DON'T HAVE PLENTY OF TIME

On the Heathrow Express into Paddington, I overhear a woman lamenting the fact that she wants to have a baby but doesn't have a partner. It's the same story that is echoed every day in corridors over water coolers, in cafes over lattes, in bars over daiquiris, and everywhere and anywhere 30-something women congregate. The woman on the train is worried that she's getting too old and will run out of time. And then, as if reading from a script, the friend delivers the lines that female friends seem genetically hardwired to deliver at times like these.

'Don't worry,' the friend says, 'you still have plenty of time. My sister's friend had a baby when she was 42, and what about Madonna, and Nicole Kidman, and Courteney Cox, and Cherie Blair?'

It's the unwritten rule of female friendship: regardless of truth or reality, our job is to make our friends feel better. We'll list examples of other people triumphing no matter how unlikely or how different their situation is and imply that if it happened to them it could happen to our friend. Why do we do it? After all, propagating false hope is surely the worst thing we can do to our friends. While we may be making our friends feel better in that very instant, we are making things worse for them in the long run.

It takes all the restraint I have not to turn around on the train and say, 'I'm sure your friend is a lovely person and wants the best for you, but don't listen to the lies she's telling you. Yes, you are getting old, and no, you don't have plenty of time. Despite what we see in the news and the glossy celebrity magazines, the chance of getting pregnant in your 40s is roughly about the same as a male underwear model reading a book: sure, it happens, just not that often.'

When it comes to our fertility, after the age of 27 it's all downhill. By our mid-30s, the fertility rates drop so dramatically it's like falling off a cliff. By 45, it's pretty much game over, unless you use somebody else's eggs. I wonder how many 40-something Hollywood stars having babies use donor eggs. When you consider the statistics – the dismal fertility rates of women over 40 – many, or even most, of these women would have had to use donor eggs. Celebrities may be able to stall the clock on the outside, but I'm yet to hear about Botox injections for ovaries. Just because you're still ovulating doesn't mean you're fertile enough to have a baby.

Even if all our equipment is in working order, it can still take years to conceive. We spend so much of our teens and 20s trying to avoid pregnancy on the quite reasonable assumption that these are our most fertile years, but when we hit our late 20s and 30s, our thinking doesn't change. Even though a decade has passed, we still assume that we're as fertile as we were at 16. The truth is it's hard to get pregnant. This is not a particularly pleasant thought, because by the time many of us get around to having babies, we don't have years – or even months – to waste.

Julie Vargo and Maureen Regan, the authors of *A Few Good Eggs*, spell it out neatly. You ovulate once a month and are fertile, give or take, for about a day. That gives you only 12 days in a whole year when you can conceive. Even for a normal couple without any fertility problems, the chance of conceiving during the month of trying is 25 per cent. That brings our twelve possible days of conception down to a lousy three days in a whole year. And that's when everything is working, when you're not too old and when you manage to coordinate yourselves to have sex at the right time.

I spent my 20s trying not to get pregnant and freaking out if I ever forgot to take a pill, or if I had gastroenteritis and may have vomited the pill up before I'd digested it. When I wasn't on the pill, I was just as anxious that the condom might split or slip off. I once almost slept with a guy who put the condom on the wrong way and then took it off, flipped it inside out and put it on the right way. I told him that we couldn't use it now because the outside of the condom had touched his dick. I was convinced that that was enough to get me pregnant. He told me that it would be fine and that I was ruining the mood. I told him that it wouldn't be fine and that having his kid would ruin my mood for the rest of my life. That relationship didn't last.

The first time I understood the fragile state of my fertility was when I was sitting in Dr Lucy's office being told that it may already be too late. I don't think I am unusually ignorant. It seems to me that most women have no idea how hard it is to conceive. In sex-education classes in school, it's implied that there is a one-to-one relationship between an unprotected shag and getting knocked up. So we go through life delaying the baby decision and foolishly believing we can pop out a baby when it's convenient. We are crippled by our ignorance and only find out the bitter truth when we are sitting in our doctor's office, when it may already be too late.

Ignorance makes us powerless. Rather than making informed and active decisions, we become passive and leave things to fate and chance. This is truly strange when you think about it. As modern women, we attempt to exert control over every other aspect of our lives – we manage our education, our careers, our finances, our personal development – yet when it comes to our fertility, we bury our heads in the sand and choose not to think about it, much less act on it, until the alarms on our biological clocks are ringing. How are we supposed to think straight when our alarms are already going off? While we are busying ourselves with our denial and clinging on to the one-in-a-million stories in which a woman in her 50s managed to get pregnant, we are wasting valuable time. We are quite possibly wasting the last couple of years, or couple of months, of our fertility.

The good news is that advances in technology and changes in laws and social attitudes have given us many more options than we had even a few years ago. I didn't realise until Dr Lucy gave me the fertility lecture that when it comes to making a baby it is the age of the embryo that matters, not the age of the mother. This means that if you're worried you are running out of time, you could freeze some embryos as a back-up plan or insurance policy in case Mr Right doesn't show up at the right time. If you decide to use them in a couple of years then they will be the age you were when you froze them. Unfortunately, the success rate of freezing unfertilised eggs is not great, which is why you would most likely have to source some sperm to make embryos and freeze those instead. I don't want to imply that becoming a single mother by choice is easy or even desirable. But if you want a baby, or think you might want one in the future, and you don't have a Chris, then surely it's an option to seriously consider and plan for.

I admit that this adds a whole layer of complexity, and the moral and ethical issues can't be underestimated. The process for collecting eggs and freezing embryos involves an expensive and invasive surgical procedure, which alone may be enough to turn you off. I'm not suggesting that this is an easy decision or even that it's the right decision. But it is a decision. We don't have to be passive spectators when it comes to our fertility.

So the next time one of our friends is worrying about her ticking clock and the absence of the man of her dreams, consider working from a different script. Rather than propagating false hope to make her feel better, why not suggest that if she really wants a baby she should start exploring her options before it's too late. Knowing what I know now, I think all women should take the time to seriously think about their fertility options at an age when they still have choices. If you are certain, in your heart of hearts, that you don't ever want kids, then so be it. Celebrate your active and deliberate choice to be childfree. But make it a choice and not the default outcome because you left it too late.

I want to deliver a lecture to the woman on the train, but I don't. I want to tell her that if she wants children in the future then she should have a plan – and a contingency plan. If Prince Charming doesn't ride into her life on schedule, or if he turns into a toad after she mentions commitment or babies, then she needs to think about writing an alternative ending to her fairy tale.

# 15

## NEVER SAY NEVER

'So are you going to get married?' my friend Stephen asks a few days later when I break the good news that Chris and I want to have a baby.

This is unexpected.

I stare at him for a moment, unable to make sense of the question. In my mind, having a baby and getting married are as unrelated as having a baby and baking a quiche. And besides, what century are we living in? 'I don't think you need to worry that our bastard child will be shunned by society,' I reply.

Obviously as part of my decision to have a baby I have factored in my relationship and commitment to Chris. I've agonised over the permanence of motherhood, so I am well aware that a child will create a bond between Chris and me for life, whether we want to be bound or not. By making a commitment to have a child, I am also, without reservation, making a commitment to Chris.

Six months ago, if you had asked me if I wanted to be with Chris for ever, I would have said, 'Only if it makes both of us happy.' And, given my belief in the impermanence of all things in life, I would think it unlikely that we would be happy together until death do us part. When the Wiccans make a marriage vow until death do us part, they are referring to the death of the love, not the people. When they marry, also known as handfasting, they pledge to stay together for as long as they are both happy in the relationship. If and when they get to the point where they are no longer happy, they break up. This makes sense to me. What's the point of staying in a marriage that makes you unhappy? Surely a successful marriage should be measured by how happy it is rather than its longevity. When people speak of a marriage that fails, I don't think of one that has broken up, I think of one in which the couple have stayed together despite no longer loving each other. Where's the achievement in two people enduring decades of bitter misery together?

I honestly believe that a big factor in a successful marriage is luck. People grow and evolve over time. Surely it's just luck when people grow and evolve in a mutually compatible direction. I'm not the person I was ten years ago. I see the world and my place in it quite differently from the way I did even a year ago, let alone a decade ago. If I had married the person I was in love with when I was 20 and had felt compelled to stay with him for life, I would be living in a world of misery now. What I wanted in a man back then is almost the antithesis of what I want in a man now. For example, the ability to consume half a bottle of tequila and still dance the Macarena doesn't even make it into my 'Top Ten Attributes I Look For in a Man' list, as it did fifteen years ago. When my tastes have changed so radically in the past, how can I possibly know what I will want 15 years from now?

This is why I don't believe in marriage. I see it as a gamble: one that is laced with social disapproval if it doesn't pay off. A broken relationship is viewed quite differently from a broken marriage. There is very little, if any, social disapproval when a relationship breaks up. When a long-term relationship breaks up, people inevitably feel sad, but when a marriage breaks up not only are they sad they are also burdened by guilt. The only difference I see between a relationship and a marriage is a declaration before church or state and having to pay for a whole lot of people to get pissed on your bar tab. I don't think the church or the state have any business getting involved in my relationships, and second cousins twice removed whose names I can't even remember can buy their own damn drinks.

When my parents' marriage broke up, I became very curious, and, I confess, quite bitter as well, about the institution of marriage. I asked all my parents' friends about their marriages to see if I could find any evidence that long-term marriage was anything but an impossible ideal. One of my mother's friends told me that she'd had hard times in her marriage, but each time they hit a bump in the road they had decided to stay together because they had too much to lose. Too much to lose! What sort of reason is that to stay together? This is not the stuff of Hallmark cards. My great-aunt said to me, 'My girl, it's not that I don't believe in marriage, it's just that my life has got much better since my husband died.'

Even penguins aren't much of an inspiration here. As any Discovery Channel wildlife expert will tell you, penguins are supposed to mate for life. But it turns out even they can't manage it. Apparently 30 per cent of penguins have affairs. And they live on ice floes for God's sake, where the opportunities for a bit of feather on the side are presumably few and far between. Even now when I think about all the long-term married couples that I know, I can think of very few who seem to be happily married. I have a hard time believing the ones who insist that they are happy. After all, I spent most of my life believing that my parents were happily married only to discover that they weren't and never had been.

I tell Stephen about all the books I've been reading about motherhood and how a happy marriage seems even more unlikely once you add children to the equation. 'A baby is a hand grenade tossed into a marriage,' I tell him, quoting Nora Ephron.

It turns out that Ephron was on to something. Some researchers pinpoint the birth of the first child as the trigger for the downward spiral of marital dissatisfaction that often ends in divorce. It's not just the early days of sleep deprivation and role adjustment when your marriage turns to shit. Oh no, it goes on for much longer than that. In their book *When Partners Become Parents: The Big Life Change for Couples*, Carolyn Pape Cowan and Philip A. Cowan write about a study in which they tracked approximately one hundred couples for five years after the birth of their first child. They found that 97 per cent of couples reported that there had been an increase in marital conflict since the birth of their child, and almost 25 per cent of couples reported that their marriage was in distress even 18 months after the bundle of joy had arrived.

I feel pretty confident that I have mounted a convincing case to support my anti-marriage position. My high-school debating teacher would have been proud. But then Stephen strikes back with his killer counter-argument. He agrees with me that divorce carries stigma and shame and also that having kids strains even the very strongest of relationships. But then he turns my words against me and says that these are the very reasons why you should get married.

'The institution of marriage is an extra safeguard that helps you stay together,' Stephen says. 'If you have a child, wouldn't you want to do everything you could to stay together for it?'

Crap. I don't have a comeback to that – or at least not one that I can convince myself of, let alone Stephen. As an adult, I was truly devastated by my parents' divorce. As a family, I doubt that we will ever recover from it. I can only imagine how much harder it would have been for me if my dad had left when I was a child. Even though I side with Dr Phil when he says that a broken home is better for children than an unhappy home, I can't bear the thought of inflicting the pain and instability of a broken home on my child. If the institution of marriage would make me try one more time or work that little bit harder before I changed the locks and pawned my wedding ring, then it's hard for me to see it as anything but a good thing.

I hate the idea that in a single sentence Stephen can reverse a belief that I have held so passionately for so many years. I've never pictured myself as married, but then again I've never pictured myself as a mother either. This is shaping up to be the year of never say never.

As soon as I say goodbye to Stephen, I phone Chris to relay our conversation. I can barely believe what I'm hearing when Chris says that he agrees with Stephen. I was expecting him to come up with the rebuttal argument I was unable to think of myself.

'If you believe in marriage,' I ask in disbelief, 'then why haven't you ever said anything about it?'

'Because you told me on our first date that you'd never get married and I believed you,' Chris says.

'So, hypothetically speaking, you'd be willing to marry me?'

'Yes, puss cat.'

That night, somewhere between 'What should we have for dinner?' and 'What do you want to do at the weekend?' Chris casually slips into the conversation, 'So do you think we should get married?'

'Not so fast,' I tell him. It's not easy to totally back flip on one of my most passionately and firmly held beliefs in less than a twelve-hour period. I need to think about it.

And when I say 'think', I mean it. I need to bring out the heavy guns. And so I return to the Vipassana meditation centre for another gruelling session of silence, isolation, hunger and physical pain. I can't get enough time off work to go for the full ten-day meditation course as I did last time, so I have to make do with a three-day course. A ten-day course is out of the question anyway, as I'm due to ovulate in five days' time. Given that abstinence and gender segregation are mandatory at the meditation centre, I think it unlikely that they would grant me a conjugal visit.

The whole point of meditation is to control your mind so that you solely focus on the physical sensations in your body. You are supposed to block out all those random thoughts that are constantly flowing through your mind, the ones that are full of self-doubt and criticism, or even the mundane ones about when you are due for a leg wax or whether or not you remembered to pack underwear. During my ten-day course, there were times when I managed to turn off the mental noise and my inner self-critic. I call it 'gagging my inner bitch'. And during those times one of two things happened: my mind was silent and I felt the most sublime sense of peace, or I had 'ah ha' moments. You know, those rare moments where everything just seems to fall into place. I had realisations that resolved issues that had been bothering me for years, and I went away feeling more peaceful, less burdened and more of a grown-up. I'm hoping the same will happen this time.

As I sit in the meditation hall for the very first meditation session on the first day, I am overcome by a desire to run from the place screaming. I remember with absolute clarity how emotionally and physically painful it was last time and can't believe I have willingly returned to do it all over again. People have told me that this is what happens when you give birth to your second child. You somehow forget that childbirth is, as Kathy Lette so eloquently puts it in *Foetal Attraction*, like 'excreting a block of flats' until the contractions start and then it's too late to do anything about it. I surrender to my three-day labour and hope that by the end of it I will have given birth to some clarity of thought.

This turns out to be an appropriate analogy, because during the three days I see mental pictures of myself as a mother. They are as clear as if I'm looking at photos, which is unusual for me because I'm not a visual person at all. I see myself cuddling a baby girl. Then I'm pushing her on a swing, helping her with her homework and even comforting her first broken heart. It's like looking forward, instead of back, at the photo album and home videos of my life. And in almost every image, I see Chris. Mostly he's in the foreground, sometimes in the background, but always there. During the nights, I lie on my hard bunk bed listening to my stomach rumbling and pondering my objections to marriage. If I am committed enough to Chris to have a child with him, a bond that can never be broken, why wouldn't I want to marry him?

As soon as I turn my mobile phone on after leaving the meditation centre, I discover an urgent message from Emma. I call her back and discover that I'm not the only one who spent the weekend contemplating marriage.

'I'm engaged,' Emma says.

I laugh and say, 'Who to?'

'To Matt,' she says.

'You're joking,' I say.

'No I'm not.'

'Yes you are.'

'I'm being serious,' she says.

'No you're not,' I say.

The conversation goes on like this for many more minutes until I have no option but to believe she's telling the truth. Does nothing in my world make sense any more? I would have sooner believed that Emma was moving to Tibet to become a Buddhist nun than that she would ever get married.

Matt took Emma away for the weekend to see the fairy penguins. As they were sitting on the beach at dusk watching the fairy penguins waddle out of the water and into their burrows, Matt told Emma that he wanted to spend the rest of his life with her. He knew it was a big step for Emma, but he said that it was what he really wanted, so he had to take the risk of asking.

'What did you say when he asked you?' I ask.

'I said "yes".'

'What, straight away? Just like that, you back flipped on one of your most firmly held beliefs?'

'Look who's talking.'

She has a point.

I am so shocked by Emma's news that I forget my manners and all social convention. I completely forget to congratulate her. So I meet up with her the next day for a coffee to offer my congratulations and further interrogate her about the decision.

She is wearing the beautiful handcrafted necklace Matt gave her when he proposed. 'What did your mum say?' I ask.

When Emma rang her mum with the news, the first thing Jenny said was, 'Oh, wonderful. That means I'm going to get grandchildren soon.'

'Is she going to get some grandchildren soon?' I ask.

Emma sighs. 'Babies are like aliens in my world. I'm a rational person and babies aren't rational. And you can't sleep, can't work, you look like shit, your brain doesn't function, your relationship turns to shit, you've got no personal time, you have to sacrifice your shoe collection, but it's the best thing you've ever done. Yeah, right.'

'You might want to sort out the baby issue before you get married,' I suggest. 'It's not something you can compromise on.'

'I know,' Emma says. 'I've got almost a year before the wedding to change my mind. I've got time up my sleeve if it comes to the crunch and I really can't do it.'

I'm not sure if she's joking or not. I'm trying to come up with something insightful and helpful to say when Emma jumps in with, 'My mum has some advice for you. She wants me to tell you that you need to have more sex.' Emma's imitation of Jenny is frighteningly accurate. 'The trouble with you girls today is that you're not having enough sex. You can't have sex once or twice and expect to make a baby. Young people today don't know how to work for things.'

If only she knew.

A couple of days later, Emma casually slips into conversation that she plans to change her name when she gets married. I shouldn't be surprised, but I am. By now I should accept that whatever people say in their 20s turns out to be crap in their 30s. But I remember the conversation as if it were yesterday when Emma told me she would never change her name. It was over ten years ago. We had skipped our lecture on macroeconomics and gone to the campus club to share a glass of the cheapest white wine on the menu. We skipped the lecture simply because we could, and the single glass of house white was the only thing we could afford. We were both wearing peasant skirts with thick belts around our hips – a bad choice for both of us. And she said to me, most emphatically, 'I'm not a piece of property; it's not like changing the name on the deeds to a house. And why shouldn't the man change his name for me?'

More than a decade later, when we can afford to have a drink each (except mine is non-alcoholic, to improve fertility), Emma revokes her stance by saying, 'Family is really important to Matt and having the same name is a symbol of family.'

'Yes, but your name used to be a symbol of your identity, and your identity is important to you,' I say.

'My view on these things now is to just go with it unless it does harm. If it's important to Matt and it's not going to do me any harm, then I'll just go with it.'

Is this what ageing is all about? Do the years of experience wear away the topsoil of our ideals so that all that remains is the hard rock of pragmatism and the desire to keep the peace?

Two weeks later, Chris and I are having dinner at our favourite cheap and cheerful Vietnamese restaurant when he produces a little box tied up with a bow. My heart skips a beat for a moment, until I realise that the box is too big to be a standard ring box. It's not a ring. It's a shiny new pink iPod. The back of the iPod is tattooed with, 'I love you, Kasey. Love Chris.' And the belly of the iPod is filled with the *Pride and Prejudice* mini-series – the Colin Firth version, of course.

'I'd really like to marry you,' Chris says. He thought proposing with a ring would freak me out. He's right. He also thought I'd like to pick my own ring. Right again.

That night we have sex. And I'm not even ovulating.

# 16

# CHRYSANTHEMUMS ARE SUCH UGLY FLOWERS

It's the sixth time my tear-streaked face has stared into the toilet and seen death. Why do I always get my period at work? Six months of 'trying' and six months of failing. For the first time, it dawns on me that perhaps it really is too late. Perhaps I'm already infertile.

I know now that when Dr Lucy told me that it might already be too late I didn't actually believe her. Why would I? I've grown up believing that everything is within my reach. I could have anything, so long as I wanted it enough and worked hard enough for it. Despite my initial ambivalence, my desire for a baby has grown exponentially with each passing month, and I'm now quite certain that I've never wanted anything more than I want a baby. And when it comes to conception sex, we've been working hard. Damn hard. I guess there was always a part of me that clung to the belief that Dr Lucy was just trying to scare me, or that somehow I was different. In my mind, somewhere deep below the surface, I believed that infertility is something that happens to other people, people who smoked too much pot and abused their bodies.

As I flush away my optimism and self-denial, I'm overcome by a sense of despair. As dramatic as this sounds, I feel as though the worst experiences in my life could not have prepared me for the devastation

I feel at this moment. I've spent almost 30 years of my life knowing for sure that I didn't want kids and the last few months knowing for sure that I do. But it isn't until this moment that I realise that I need them. Just like my friend Danielle, I need a child with every fibre of my being, and the thought that my body simply isn't up to the job is too much to bear. I feel angry, inadequate, guilty and self-indulgent all at once. The emotions are so raw I feel like I'm about to burst. At the same time, I'm consumed by a sense of emptiness – a void so deep that not even my self-pity can fill it.

I fear I'll never get to live out the fantasy of walking into the lounge carrying a pregnancy stick emblazoned with that magical second line as if it were a trophy. It's the fantasy where Chris will embrace me and tell me he loves me while he bats away the tear of joy that has crept into the corner of his eye. I will never be able to tell my mum that I'm giving her a grandchild, and Chris will never be able to tell his parents either. All of them will be denied the pleasure and delight of hearing this news, because of me, because I'm broken. My infertility is not just my disappointment and my heartache; it's Chris's and our families' as well.

Mother's Day is just around the corner, and the mere thought of it is enough to sink me even lower. Telling myself that Mother's Day is a commercial conspiracy between Hallmark and the Chrysanthemum Growers Association doesn't make me feel any better. I allow more waves of self-pity to wash over me and shed a tear for the bunch of ugly weeds – chrysanthemums are such ugly flowers – I'll never be given. It doesn't matter how great the rest of my life is. And it is great. When it comes to the good things in life, I've already got more than my fair share. But this doesn't console me. I'm incapable of focusing on what I do have because I am totally blinded by what I don't have, what I may never have.

I sneak out of the toilet hoping that no one will notice I've been in there for almost an hour. I've reapplied my make-up, but there isn't much I can do about my red-rimmed eyes. I've almost made it through the foyer and back to my desk when I bump into Sarah. Sarah is a colleague who I haven't seen for ages, for months, in fact. Now that I see her sitting on a couch in the foyer rocking a baby in her arms, it dawns on me that I haven't seen her since, let me see . . . That's it: since she went on maternity leave.

Oh, for fuck's sake. Is this some elaborate conspiracy that everyone else is in on apart from me? It's the perfect picture: the baby is sleeping peacefully and Sarah is looking like a fulfilled, blissful yummy mummy. Everywhere I look there are bloody babies and pregnant women, taunting me and constantly reminding me of what I can't have. I've started to notice the signs on public transport that indicate priority seating for the elderly and pregnant women. Even the signs are pregnant. The other day on the news I heard that even the fucking elephant at the fucking zoo is fucking pregnant.

I hurry past Sarah, hoping she won't notice me. No such luck. She calls me over and introduces me to Oliver. He's perfect. Even the rolls of fat on his chubby knees are perfect. 'Congratulations,' I say, choking over the word.

Sarah misinterprets my awkwardness as a dislike for babies. 'I used to feel that way about babies too,' she says. 'But then I accidentally missed one pill and look what happened.' She kisses Oliver on the forehead and beams with delight. 'He's the best mistake I ever made. You should do it, Kasey. Motherhood is the best thing ever.'

Could this get any worse? She gets pregnant after a bout of absentmindedness, while Chris and I have been having so much sex that we're getting chafing. Rather than pointing out the fundamental injustice of life in general, I change the subject from babies by asking what she's doing here. One of the account directors has asked her to come in for a meeting and she suspects he's going to ask her to come back to work early. Sarah says she's going to decline the offer and confides that she doesn't think she'll ever come back.

'There's nothing in the world I'd rather be than a mother,' she says. 'But I won't tell the company that.'

As if on cue, Oliver blinks open his sleepy eyes and shoots me a toothless grin. Sarah holds him out to me. 'Here, hold him,' she says.

'See how good it feels.' I shake my head and step back as if her child is diseased. I feel rude, but I can't bring myself to hold him. In fact, I can barely look at him. I hurriedly say goodbye and rush straight back into the toilets, holding it together just long enough to get into the privacy of the cubicle. Once inside, the tears start to flow again. I don't fight them. I just sit there crying my eyes out, feeling miserable and pissed off. I try to make myself feel better by thinking that 'Sarah may have Oliver, but at least I still have a waist', but it is of little comfort.

Why is it that Sarah can have a baby 'by mistake' when I can't manage it even though there is more sex going on in my bedroom than the busiest brothel in town? Why is it that there are approximately 225 million pregnancies in the world every year and I can't even manage just one? What's worse is that it's estimated that over a third of these pregnancies are unwanted. I know there is no justice or fairness when it comes to fertility. But, damn it, there bloody well should be.

As the wave of emotion subsides, I realise that I'm genuinely happy for Sarah. It's a weird feeling to be happy for somebody else yet completely devastated for myself. I think of my twin brother Wesley, who has a gorgeous little girl. They live in Canada, so I haven't met her yet. I haven't seen any photos or heard any news about my little niece for months, ever since I told him about my infertility issues, in fact. I know my brother is emailing photos and home videos of her to everyone in the family except me. He is sensitive and considerate, so I'm sure he has omitted me from the email list with the very best of intentions. But somehow it makes me feel worse.

What happens when such a basic need isn't met? Are you condemned to live an unfulfilled life? Or can you re-create yourself into a person who has different needs – into a person who can be both infertile and happy all at once?

Instead of returning to my desk, I tell the receptionist that I have an urgent teleconference and ask her to book a meeting room for me. I also tell her that I can't be disturbed. Once inside, I phone Emma.

'Do you know of any women who are childless and genuinely happy?' I ask.

'Sure,' she says, and then she lists the names of some of her 20-something friends and colleagues.

'But they don't count,' I insist. When I was 20-something, I was childless and genuinely happy too. 'Do you know of any childless women who are past their childbearing years and are genuinely not regretful that they didn't have or couldn't have kids?'

Emma thinks about it for a moment and then sounds surprised by her own response. 'I can't think of any,' she says. 'But I can name a heap who are regretful and neurotic.'

'That's not the answer I want to hear,' I say.

'That's not the answer I want to give,' she says as the realisation of what we're potentially facing hits her. 'I don't want to be miserable and fucked up later in life if I don't have kids.'

A psychologist once told me that having children is a necessary life stage for women. He quoted the legendary psychologist Erik Erikson's life-stage development theory. The psychologist told me that if a childless 40-something woman presents in his clinic, he knows that she's going to have serious issues that will take years to work through. At the time, I didn't want to believe it. I hate the idea that there is only one path to happiness. And now that I'm staring childlessness in the face, I really, really, really don't want to believe it.

I tell Emma that she needs to go on the prowl for happily childless middle-aged women, and I will do the same. I need to know that they exist. I need to know that regardless of what happens, I will be able to write myself a happy ending.

I don't know if it's just the circles that I mix in, but I don't know of many middle-aged women who don't have children. In fact, out of all the people I know, I can only think of one. Unfortunately, she's travelling at the moment, and it seems bad manners to send her an email out of the blue to ask if she's happy and whether or not she considers herself to be neurotic. If I am to ask this of anyone, the very least I can do is buy them a drink.

I send an email out to my friends asking if they know of a 50-something happily childless woman who would be willing to speak to me. No one can help me. Eventually I meet Liz, a 50-something career counsellor, at a book club, and she agrees to catch up with me again so I can quiz her on her life choices. We meet in a funky little cafe that looks deliberately and tastefully run-down, the kind that hangs the work of local artists on the walls and only sells organic produce. I feel like I'm observing Liz in her native habitat. She dresses young and edgy for her age, without looking like mutton. And she's well groomed and attractive without looking made-up. I'd bet a hundred quid that she has a pot of fresh herbs growing on her windowsill.

Liz tells me her decision to remain childless is a choice and that she's happy. She assures me that her extended independent-woman phase is not at all boring or vacuous. At the ripe old age of 16, Liz decided she never wanted kids, and with the window of her fertility now firmly closed, she is certain that she doesn't regret the decision. She wanted a life full of travel and study instead. She confides that her desire to remain childless was heavily influenced by her own childhood.

Liz's parents grew up in the Depression. Her mother was awarded a scholarship to finish her high-school education but was unable to accept it because she had to go out to work. Then she had children and was never able to finish her education.

'She never got over it,' Liz tells me. 'She died at 85, and she always resented it. She suffered from depression because she didn't live the life she wanted. She always felt that life had let her down.'

Because her mother's life ambitions were thwarted by marriage and children, Liz didn't have a very happy childhood. 'I wasn't abused as a child, it was more neglect.' To make matters worse, her father desperately wanted sons and ended up with only daughters. 'I was the fourth disappointment,' she says.

'I always knew that I didn't have the stuff to be a good mother. I didn't want to impose that on another human being,' she says. 'I have seen two of my three sisters have kids and they were both dismal failures as parents. Both their marriages split up and the kids are very troubled. The kids haven't learned to be independent or considerate. My parents weren't good at it and neither were my sisters.'

At twenty-one, Liz married an industrial chemist who died six months later. If he'd lived, she probably would have ended up having kids. 'We do things because that's what society expects,' she says. 'The shutters go down and we do things without thinking.

'Some people say that I'm selfish for not having children. I think it's their own defensiveness about the choices they made. I think there is a hint of jealousy behind their accusation because they want the life I've got.' It's not that Liz doesn't like kids; she loves her nieces and nephews and her friends' kids, and she worked as a nanny in London for a while. 'I love kids, but I just don't want my own.'

For a brief period when she was 37, she felt differently. She says her hormones kicked in and she wanted a baby. 'It was ghastly,' she says. 'It was such a struggle, because my biological impulse was so strong.' The battle was even harder because she was dating a man at the time who would have happily had kids with her. 'But I forced myself to make the decision not to have them, and once I'd put the stake in the ground and made the firm decision that this was my hormones talking and not what I really wanted, then the tension and energy could dissipate and I could get on with the rest of my life.'

I tell Liz about Erik Erikson's theory that all people have the desire to nurture and influence and therefore if we don't have kids we end up being unfulfilled and fucked up. She says that she definitely has the need to nurture, but rather than nurturing a child, she's nurturing herself. 'I'm discovering a broader, deeper me and coming to grips with my own strengths, both personally and professionally,' she says. 'It's self-indulgent, but it's also a privilege to devote my time to me, my life and the world around me. Maybe my metaphorical baby is still to come, or perhaps the baby I'm raising is me. I'm developing me and exploring my own potential.'

Liz's nurturing side is also being fulfilled through her work as a career counsellor. She specialises in working with people who have been made redundant. She helps them deal with the emotional turmoil of losing their jobs, to work out what they really want to do next and then helps with the mechanics of getting a job, such as CV preparation and interview skills.

Most of her friends have adult children. I ask her if it was an issue when her friends' kids were younger. Did she feel excluded or neglected?

'No. It was never an issue. I didn't ever feel like I wasn't in the club. I was like Aunty Lizzy without actually being Aunty Lizzy.

'Women who choose not to have children must have a strong sense of self-confidence and self-love, to know that they are worthy people and complete women. There is a tidal wave of social pressure to have kids. The woman who can state without flinching that she chose not to be a mother has found great strength within herself to face that prejudice.'

Liz isn't worried about being childless and alone in old age.

'This was the main reason my mother had kids,' Liz says, 'and I've seen first-hand the manipulation and nastiness that transpired as the result. It's really quite ugly. I'm responsible for me. I think a parent's job is to bring up kids to be independent and responsible for looking after themselves. They shouldn't be raising carers for their own old age.'

Liz says she's seen what her friends have gone through in caring for declining and dying parents, the pain and anguish it caused. 'I think a lot of older people are not making the right decisions at the right times, and the burden then falls to their children to make the decisions about where they are going to live and how they are going to be cared for. I don't have any expectations that anyone will look after me when I get older.'

Liz plans to sell her house and move into a retirement village. She has given one of her friends the power of medical attorney and the friend has been given strict instructions that if Liz is rendered unconscious and can't make a full recovery then she doesn't want to be resuscitated. The only concern Liz has about her old age is being sufficiently financially secure to fund those last few years of her life. But she points out that having children is not necessarily a safeguard against poverty in old age anyway.

I ask her if she had her time over would she have had kids?

'I made the right decision,' she says emphatically. 'Even though I have had hard times, I am thankful for the life I've had. I really like the life I am living right now. I have fantastic friends; I am engaged with my broader family. I'm the organiser for family get-togethers. I can go away when I want, and do courses. I'm certainly alone, but I don't feel lonely. Only occasionally do I miss having someone to be around and hang out with.'

As I say goodbye to Liz, I am thinking about the baby switch: the one that flicks on in your 30s that makes you crazy with baby lust – the one I'm dealing with at the moment. Even though Liz has been certain all her life that she didn't want kids, she still had to battle the baby switch. But she didn't view the switch as an indication of a biological necessity to breed but more like a disease she caught and fortunately recovered from without any life-long scars. It comforts me to think that just as quickly and intensely as the baby switch can flick on, it can also flick off.

My friend Cathy tells a similar story. Cathy desperately wanted a baby and tried to conceive via IVF for years. By the time her 40s had crept up on her, she eventually accepted that she would never be able to have a baby. I had always assumed she was still, and would forever be, deeply wounded by her childlessness. In fact, if she had told me that she no longer craved a baby and she was happily childfree I wouldn't have believed her. However, she surprises me when I phone her for a chat and she tells me that she's had 'the most stressful week of my life'. Her period was late, her breasts were sore and her tummy felt swollen. It dawned on her that the impossible had happened – that she could, in fact, be pregnant. It was too early to pee on a stick. As a conception-sex expert, she is well aware that you need to wait ten days after conception before you can test for pregnancy.

Cathy endured a few very nervous and very long days until her period arrived, and during that time she realised that she didn't actually want a baby any more. 'I swear,' she says. 'I really didn't want to be pregnant. I've never been so relieved when my period arrived.' When Cathy's desire for a baby was taken out of the world of hypotheticals and 'what ifs' and subjected to a real-world test, it became clear that her baby switch had gone off and her life has moved on. Cathy is busy building a business, studying and travelling. The space in her life that she used to think could only be filled by a child has been filled by other things.

Liz and Cathy's stories console me a little bit. Clearly it is possible to be both well functioning and childless.

# 17

## NUNS ARE SCARY

I can't believe I'm marrying a Catholic. In fact, I can't believe I'm marrying a Christian. It's not that I have anything against them. On the contrary, I always worry that they'll have something against me. My first serious relationship was with a lovely Christian boy. There were many reasons why this relationship was never going to last, the most obvious being that I loved him far more than he loved me. But when he told his parents he had a girlfriend, the first question they asked was 'Is she a Christian?' This was a deal-breaker for them. While they were hospitable enough to grant a temporary access visa to their family, I would never qualify for citizenship.

After that experience, I figured I'd stick to atheists or agnostics when it came to dating. This was made easier by the section on Internet dating websites in which people declared their religion. I instantly discounted anybody who said they were religious. So how did I end up with Chris the Catholic? He sneakily left that box blank. It wasn't until our third date, when I was already head over heels for him, that he confessed. He claims that it was a fortunate oversight and he simply forgot to tick the box on the website. It was fortunate indeed, because if he had checked the box I would never have met him for that first drink after work, which turned into dinner, which turned into goodnight coffee, which turned into the present discussion about whether or not we should get married in a church.

When I was younger, I was so principled in my decisions that I was a complete pain in the arse. Things were simply right or wrong; there were no messy shades of grey and no compromises. Back then I would refuse to set foot in a Catholic church as long as there was rampant AIDS in Africa and paedophile priests being protected. I do still condemn the Catholic church for the obscene role it's played in these crimes, but I now realise that not all Catholics are evil and that refusing to enter a church isn't going to right either of these wrongs. Now I value harmony over principle. Getting married in the tiny sandstone church that Chris's parents married in 40 years earlier will mean the world to him and his parents. And I actually don't care where I get married. I have no childhood wedding fantasy that I need to realise. So when I agree to marry in the church, I consider it more as a gift to Chris's family than a sell-out of my principles. I'm also quite chuffed that the Catholics will have me, although, as Chris is quick to point out, the Catholics will take anybody these days.

It's not until later that I realise that getting married in a Catholic church comes with a catch. It's called a marriage preparation course. I'm truly terrified of sitting in front of a nun, discussing our relationship. In fact, I'm terrified of nuns full stop, regardless of what we are discussing. I've seen the movie *The Magdalene Sisters*, in which the nuns lock up girls who get pregnant out of wedlock and force them to spend all day, every day washing sheets. For these girls their pregnancies were accidents. How much laundry will I have to do if I deliberately get pregnant out of wedlock? Emma puts my mind at ease. 'Regardless of your marital status,' she says, 'if you have a baby you'll spend all day doing laundry anyway.'

I'm so intimidated by all the pomp and ceremony of Catholicism that when Chris and I walk into the church for our ridiculously early weekend appointment I am reduced to an insecure schoolgirl who's been summoned to the principal's office. Will the nun be able to tell just by looking at me that I'm not a virgin? Will she know that I occasionally like to pepper my speech with words like 'shit' and 'fuck'?

We are met at the door of the church by Marjorie. I actually don't know if this is her name, but it should be. Anyone with a perfectly sculpted grey bob and wearing a lilac twinset, grey slacks and sensible pewter shoes ought to be called Marjorie.

Marjorie turns out to be a parish volunteer. She explains that she will administer the test, a multiple-choice questionnaire, which we will complete in separate rooms. The test will then be sent to head office to be collated and analysed. I'm not sure if I'm imagining a type of dodgy love computer you'd expect to see in the Chief's office in *Get Smart* or a knitting circle of middle-aged women analysing the results. Either way, I'm suspicious. Marjorie then introduces us to Sister Catherine, a stern-looking nun who will discuss our test results with us.

As I pick up my pencil to begin the test, Marjorie tells me that there are no right or wrong answers, so I just need to answer honestly. What a load of bullshit. Oh, crap, am I allowed to say 'bullshit' in a church, even if it's silently to myself?

Recruiters and human-resources people always give the 'there are no right or wrong answers' line when they are administering personality tests, and everyone knows that some answers are right enough to get you the job and other answers are wrong enough to get your application put in the 'do not hire' tray. I wonder if the Catholic tests work the same way.

I don't know what I was expecting on the test, but I'm taken aback by questions like 'Are you nervous about your future husband seeing you naked?' Holy crap! Does the church actually expect people not to have sex before marriage? Oh no, I said 'crap'. And to make matters worse, I added the word 'holy'. Is that sacrilegious? Have I just earned myself another demerit point for thinking bad language or will 'crap' be lumped with 'bullshit' in a big overarching demerit?

There are a few more questions like the naked one that clearly show that the church is out of touch with society. But I must admit that the majority of the questions are relevant, practical and thought-provoking. There are questions about what I value, how I manage money, how I deal with conflict: issues that should be discussed prior to getting married. Then I come to the questions about children, and my heart sinks. I read the question 'How will you feel if your husband is unable to have children?' and think about Chris sitting in the other room answering how he'll feel if his wife can't have kids. When all of this baby talk began, Chris told me that he wanted me more than kids. But my desire for a baby has grown so much over the past few months. Surely his has grown to the same degree. Who could blame him for preferring a fertile wife? I've read that in some cultures barrenness is sufficient grounds for divorce, or that a marriage isn't even formalised until a child is a toddler. What's the point in the relationship continuing if it doesn't produce a healthy child?

I don't believe in soulmates, and I certainly don't believe that love conquers all. I think there are very concrete and practical factors that make a relationship succeed or fail. More than anything, I believe that both halves of the couple have to be on the same page. They have to want the same things, or, at the very least, want mutually compatible things. Having children is something that you can't compromise on or substitute for something else. It worries me that the sum total of my other attributes will not be enough to compensate for my infertility.

I ask Chris about this as soon as we leave the church. I need to get it all out in the open, because if he wants children more than he wants me then I need to know and I need to know now.

'You know the question about how you'd feel if your partner is infertile?' I try to sound casual, but my voice is quivering.

'I'd be sad,' Chris says. 'I'd be really sad, but I don't think you are infertile. I still think we can do it.'

'Be realistic,' I say. 'What happens if I can't have a baby?'

'I think you can,' he says.

I love his optimism, but he's missing my point. 'But if I can't,' I insist, 'will you still want to marry me?'

'Yes, puss cat.'

He answers too quickly, and it makes me suspicious. 'I'm being serious,' I say. 'I want you to really think about it. If having a baby is a prerequisite for our happy marriage then let's deal with it now and not in ten years' time when your firm-fleshed, fertile secretary looks more appealing than your barren wife.'

'I love you, Kasey,' he says. 'And I want to marry you, no matter what.'

These are the sweetest words I've ever heard, and I use them to bolster my courage and suppress my cynicism a week later as we knock on Sister Catherine's door to talk about our test results. Although I can't help but mutter, 'What can a nun tell us about relationships? She's never had one.'

'No,' Chris says. 'But she's observed plenty and spent her life supporting people through the ups and downs of their relationships.'

It's 8 p.m. and Sister Catherine is wearing her civvies when she greets us at the door of her house. Out of her veil she looks more like your average granny than a stern laundry-enforcer. The smell of sausages is wafting in the air, and I'm comforted by the realisation that nuns eat dinner like everybody else. I guess that she's in her mid-70s, although I suppose a vow of poverty would mean she couldn't afford moisturisers and exfoliants, so perhaps she's younger than she looks.

We are guided past all the Mary prints, statues and ornaments into a sitting room where Sister Catherine offers us a drink. I figure a gin and tonic is out of the question, so I ask for a cup of tea instead.

We begin the discussion with an awkward moment. Sister Catherine asks Chris why he only completed two-thirds of the questionnaire. Did he deliberately refuse to answer any of the questions about living together and domestic responsibilities? Chris laughs and says that it wasn't until later that he realised there was a back page of the test. Sister Catherine looks relieved and says that she was unsure how to broach the subject, in case he was trying to hide something from me. She says to Chris, 'You have a PhD, don't you?' Then she shakes her head with a wry smile and says, 'The more educated people are, the less practical they become.' After that I can't help but like her.

We spend most of the time talking about finances and money management, because, as Sister Catherine says, 'All the studies show that money, and views about money, are the key to a healthy relationship and compatibility.' She has a refreshingly down-to-earth attitude to relationships, and the more we talk the more I realise that she's a very practical, no-bullshit kind of woman. So when she asks me how I feel about Catholicism, I decide to be honest with her.

'The Catholics have got a lot of bad press over the years,' I say. And before I can continue, she jumps in and says, 'Yes we have, dear, and for the most part we've deserved it.' She admits that terrible things have been done in the name of Catholicism and that this has presented challenges with her own faith. Then she says, 'Spiritual compatibility is far more important than having the same religion.'

I'm not sure what she means, so I ask her to clarify.

'Spirituality is about your values and beliefs, not the rituals you follow. I can see here that you have the same values. You're very compatible.'

As we go to leave, Sister Catherine hugs us and says, 'I'm not worried at all about you two. You'll do very well together. Sometimes I read the test results and they're so conflicting I wonder if the couple has even met before they come to see me. It amazes me that people will decide to get married without having discussed such fundamental issues.'

Back in the car, Chris says, 'I told you nuns are cool.'

And I have to admit, Sister Catherine is pretty cool.

# 18

# PREVIEW OF MENOPAUSE

When Emma suggests we go wedding-dress shopping, I burst out laughing. I know this is what brides do. It's just that I never expected either of us would ever be a bride, let alone both of us at the same time. I tell Emma that I'm happy to shop for her dress, but I don't want to shop for mine. However, I can't imagine why Emma would need my help. She has a natural sense of style that I will never have, even if I spent a lifetime trying to cultivate it. As it turns out, she doesn't need my help. In her typical no-nonsense manner, she's ordered two dresses from an up-market department store in the US. She'll pick the one she likes and send the other back. Her suggestion is to go shopping for my dress.

But I can't face it. Everything in my life has been reduced to the question about my fertility. Wedding-dress shopping is no different. When I walk down the aisle in seven months' time, I would love to do it with a waddle and an enormous bulging belly. Pregnant brides are so sexy. But I'd feel foolish and deluded looking for a wedding gown to accommodate such a belly. I'm infertile, for fuck's sake! The thought of buying a gown without room for a belly reduces me to tears. If Dr Lucy is to be believed, if I'm not pregnant by the time of my wedding it really will be game over.

Emma asks if Chris and I have thought about adopting. She reads the ambivalence on my face and says, 'Hopefully you won't need to, but don't you think you should consider it as a back-up plan?' It's a sensible suggestion, but I don't want to. I think about it for a minute and then realise the shocking truth: I don't want *a* baby, I only want *our* baby. I want a product of Chris and me. I'm not sure what this says about me, but I'm pretty sure it can't be good. Does this make me narcissistic or vain? Probably both. Does it mean that I don't really want a baby; rather I am seeking an extension of myself? I don't want to think about the answer to that question, so I tell Emma about Wendy.

Wendy and I worked together about five years ago. Her baby switch flicked on one day, surprising her and delighting her husband, Dan. Dan had been clucky for years, but Wendy was quite sure she didn't want kids until the day she realised she did. Familiar story. As far as they knew, neither of them had any fertility issues, but they didn't care if their baby was biologically theirs or adopted. At the same time as Wendy coming off the pill, they also put their names down to adopt. This surprised me at the time, because I always viewed adoption as the last resort. Clearly I was wrong. You might think that it was noble of them to put their names down to adopt, but the couples they met during the adoption registration course didn't see it that way. The infertile couples were outraged that Wendy and Dan were taking up a place on the adoption list when they were able to have their own children. The infertile couples on the list figured that people sit on the adoption list for years, so how dare fertile couples clog up the system when they could possibly have a baby the easy way. In the end, Wendy and Dan withdrew from the list and they now have three biological children.

When Chris walks through the front door a couple of hours later, I'm sitting on the couch flicking through a magazine for pregnant brides and eating a block of chocolate. I tell Chris about Emma's suggestion to go wedding-dress shopping. Chris does what he always does when he doesn't have a ready answer. He makes me a cup of tea.

He brings me a steaming cup of English Breakfast and settles down on the couch next to me. Even though I know the answer, I bring up the IVF subject again in the hope that months of fruitless fucking will have changed his mind. They haven't. Chris still firmly believes that we can conceive a child the old-fashioned way.

Dr Lucy sees it differently. I'm seeing her again for a routine post-surgery check-up to see if the endometriosis is growing back. It is, and this makes my chances of conceiving even worse than they were before. She says that if we won't start IVF then I should at least start taking fertility drugs. The drugs cause your body to ovulate multiple eggs each month rather than the standard one egg. With more eggs hanging out in your fallopian tubes, there's a greater chance that the sperm will bump into one.

Lucy does a good job of managing my expectations by informing me that my chances of conceiving are still very low because my eggs will still be second-rate and my fallopian tubes still have blockages. When I ask her about the side effects of the drugs, she replies, 'Twins, maybe triplets, maybe quads.' She says it so flippantly, as if it's no big deal, but to me having two or three or four babies at once is a very big deal. I'm a twin, and my mother has told me more times than I can count that having twins was the hardest experience of her life. This was made even worse by the fact that she had a two year old to care for as well. She says that in the beginning she couldn't even leave the house. Ever. She was so busy that the cup of tea my dad made her before he went to work was still sitting on the bench, untouched, when he walked through the door that evening. Apparently it was years before she was able to sleep through the night without interruption.

Given that I'm not even certain that I'm cut out to mother one baby, the idea of mothering multiples scares the hell out of me. The other side effects of the drugs look good in comparison to twins: hot flushes, mood swings and being overly emotional. Essentially it's a dress rehearsal for menopause.

Dr Lucy prescribes me another drug, which is supposed to improve my egg quality. The side effect of this one is nausea, making it a dress rehearsal for pregnancy.

I take Dr Lucy's prescriptions, but I'm unsure whether or not I'll actually fill them. If I'm going to do anything that could result in conceiving quads, it seems only fair that I discuss it with Chris first. We decide that the risk of multiple births is too great, so we agree that I'll start taking the egg-quality drug and leave the prescription for the fertility drug in the cupboard.

When I'm at the pharmacy collecting my prescription another wave of inadequacy washes over me. Well, actually, it crashes down on me and pummels me into the carpet. I know it's not rational, and I also know it's not helpful, but rationality is no match for emotion. These pills are a symbol of my greatest failure: greater than when I came last in my school's cross-country race, greater than when I failed woodwork class and greater than when my IQ test revealed I was in the bottom 5 per cent of the population when it came to special concepts. This is a failure of my womanhood, of what my body is designed to do. There is no chocolate in sight, so I grab a bag of jelly beans off the counter and tell the pharmacist that I'll take them too. She looks horrified.

'Are these for you?' she asks. She looks at my pills and then at the jelly beans. 'You really shouldn't be eating sugar in your condition,' she says. 'As a diabetic, this is the last thing you should be eating.'

'I'm not a diabetic,' I tell her.

She looks confused. 'Well then, what are these for?' she says, holding up the pills.

I should tell her that it's none of her damn business, that being able to recite the back of a box of pills doesn't qualify her to dispense pharmaceutical advice or make her a medical professional, so she should drop the pretence and just sell me the tablets. But thankfully I don't. She's just doing her job, after all. Instead I look around the pharmacy sheepishly to make sure there isn't anybody I know in the store and then whisper, 'They are to improve my egg quality.'

'Your what? Your eggs?' she says with the discretion and subtlety of an exploding horse.

I point at my ovaries.

'Oh,' she exclaims as if I'm hard of hearing and need each word loudly enunciated for me. 'I didn't know these were used for treating infertility.'

'Well, now you do. And so does everyone else in the store,' I snap back as I throw the money at her, grab my barren-woman pills and comfort jelly beans and run out.

Dr Lucy didn't lie about the side effects. Six hours after popping the pills, I have my head in the toilet bowl. I feel like death. Chris brings me a glass of water, and when I'm finished he cleans the toilet so it's ready for the next time. This becomes a ritual as the nausea continues relentlessly, day after day. Before long, people start commenting on how much weight I'm losing. I lie and tell them I'm trying to lose a couple of kilos before my wedding. What's one more lie in the endless web of deceit and subterfuge that is infertility?

One morning on the way to work I'm overcome by a wave of nausea. Stuck in the car, crawling along in peak-hour traffic, I know what's coming and there's nothing I can do about it. I'm about to vomit out the window when I spot a shopping bag on the floor of the car. Keeping one hand on the steering wheel and one eye on the road, I lunge to the floor on the passenger side and grab the bag. I've always been good at multitasking, but who knew it was possible to drive and vomit at the same time? Well, OK, 'drive' might be stretching it. The horns of impatient commuters are blaring all around me as I vomit mostly into the bag and partly onto my skirt.

At the first opportunity, I turn around and make my way home, holding on to the bag of vomit all the way. I can't go to work. I can't face the day, so I crawl into bed and wallow in self-pity until well into the afternoon. During my wallowing, I decide that it's time to take the fertility drug. And so begins my sneak preview of menopause.

All the weight that I lost from the nausea seems to return overnight. My ample D cup has turned into a 'they-must-be-fake' G cup. I wake up in the middle of the night dripping with sweat, kicking off the covers and stripping off my pyjamas. I have never been so hot in my life, and it's the middle of winter. When I turn on the air conditioner in the car to its coldest setting, Chris pats me on the knee and says through chattering teeth, 'You'll be OK, puss cat.'

Two weeks after performing my driving-and-vomiting trick, I'm having dinner with friends and am unable to disguise a hot flush. I'm the only one in the restaurant wearing short sleeves, but the sweat is still running down my face and dripping onto the table. Everyone stares at me. Emma gives me a knowing wink across the table and says, 'That must be one hot curry you're eating.'

I start drawing unwanted attention to myself at work too. When my account director tells me that we lost an account because I convinced a client that it was better to use an internal person rather than hire consultants, my eyes well with tears. Professionally, I know I have done the right thing. It would have been unethical for me to have advised him to use consultants just so my company could make some money. Under normal circumstances I would have made my case to the account director without remorse, but at this moment I can't decide if I want to curl up into the foetal position and beg for forgiveness or go postal and kill everybody in sight for having my judgement questioned. Feeling vulnerable, emotional and so angry that both sharp and blunt implements should be stored well out of my reach, I decide to finish early and go home.

The perverse thing about this combination of drugs is that with the nausea, mood swings, weight gain and perspiration problems, I have never felt more unattractive, unsexy and unwilling to have sex. I feel like a beached whale with anger-management issues and the libido of a discarded sock. There's no point to any of this if I'm not having sex. Just as I have to force myself to swallow the drugs every day knowing they will make me feel terrible, I now have to force myself to have sex. And this in turn throws another log onto the burning fire of my infertility guilt. I'm not even married yet and already I'm not wanting to have sex. I can only imagine how emasculating this must be for Chris.

# 19

# PROOF THAT GOD IS A MAN

A month later, we are back at Dr Lucy's office to monitor how my body is responding to the drugs. Sensing my emotional fragility, Chris comes along to the appointment with me. I try not to notice all the happy pregnant women in the waiting room, but I can't help it. I'm staring at their lovely round bellies with such longing I'm like a dog drooling over a bone.

Dr Lucy scans my ovaries with her dildo doppelgänger, and things are not good. The endometriosis has returned with a vengeance and it's doubtful that the affected ovary is functioning at all. Dr Lucy's light, jovial manner disappears and is replaced by a sternness that I've not seen before. 'Six months ago you had one and a half ovaries,' she says. 'Now you've only got one. Next time you come to see me you may have none. How much longer are you going to wait before you start IVF?'

The penny drops and I see a flicker of alarm cross Chris's face. It's the first time I've ever seen this expression from him. I don't just mean since our relationship became shrouded in the grimy cloak of infertility: I've never seen him look this way. His trademark optimism is gone as he turns to me and says, 'I think we should do it.'

'Really?' I ask, shocked at Chris's back flip. Dr Lucy is a persuasive woman, but I didn't for a moment think she'd be capable of changing Chris's mind about IVF. Chris nods.

'It's your body, so it has to be your decision. But if it's the only way for us to have a baby, then I'd like to give it a try.'

'OK,' I say. It's feels like such an inadequate response to this monumental decision. I want to say so much more. I want to acknowledge that back flipping on such a firmly held belief must be a big deal for him. I want to tell him how much I love him for his open-mindedness, pragmatism and desire to have a baby with me. And I want to shake him and ask why I had to take all those bloody vomit pills if we were going to end up doing bloody IVF anyway. I just don't want to say it all in front of Dr Lucy.

An immediate sense of relief washes over me. I'm relieved that we are about to 'do' something and end the months of hopelessly treading water, hoping for a miracle. I'm also relieved that our days of conception sex are over. To my dismay, Dr Lucy tells me to keep taking the vomit-inducing pills to improve my egg quality. The good news is that my womb looks fine, so our only challenge will be getting a decent egg. Based on my age and egg issues, Dr Lucy calculates our success rate to be 23 per cent. It's not great, but it's a lot better than many women. Apparently acupuncture can improve our success rate further. A 2008 study published in the *British Medical Journal* found that acupuncture can increase IVF success rates by up to 65 per cent.

'We used to think they were all crazy,' Dr Lucy says. 'But the evidence suggests that they're not, so we've had to open our minds to it.'

Chris, who hasn't been allowed to wank for months, for fear of wasting his precious sperm, is handed a permission slip signed by Dr Lucy along with a little jar. It's probably the first and last time that he will be told to wank on medical advice. 'You'll need to go to one of the labs listed on the back of the referral to provide a sample,' Dr Lucy says. We tell her that Chris has already done a sperm test at home, but for some reason Dr Lucy wants to verify Chris's sperm count and quality with her own test.

Chris books in for his wanking appointment and shows up the next day at the allotted time. He is sent off to a special little room with a red vinyl couch, a pile of magazines that only just pass the censor's eye and a TV with hardcore pornography on a loop. Chris grabs the remote control and flicks over to another channel. More hardcore porn. It occurs to him that one of the free-to-air channels is broadcasting the Pope delivering a sermon for World Youth Day. So at the very moment the Pope is delivering his message of hope to the faithful, Chris is watching Candi in a crotchless G-string giving some guy a blow job. Wondering how many Hail Marys he's incurring, he sits down on the protective mat covering the couch and gets to work.

A couple of days later, an envelope arrives from the IVF clinic. It contains a folder full of glossy brochures and a price list. There's a price for a standard IVF cycle where they collect the eggs, fertilise the embryos in a Petri dish and stick one up you. Or you can pay extra to get the sperm injected into the egg rather than relying on its own navigational abilities, and extra again if you'd like the embryo genetically tested before it's implanted. There's even an option to have your egg fertilised in a Petri dish carved by Tibetan monks and infused with rare and exotic plant oils originally used by Mayan Indians. OK, I made that last one up. But there are a heap of other options on the list that I don't even understand. The list is like something you'd see at a day spa with an infinite array of services and treatments.

Except this is not like choosing between a salt scrub and the hot-rock massage, this is about conceiving a child. I burst into tears when I read the price list. It's not supposed to be like this. Making a baby is supposed to be intimate and sacred, not a crass commercial endeavour.

Tucked inside the envelope is an invitation to a group counselling session about IVF. A group session! Yet another slap in the face to remind me that making our baby is no longer a private act between Chris and me. They say it takes a village to raise a baby. Since when did the village get involved in the process of making the baby as well?

An anxious knot forms in the pit of my stomach two days before the counselling session and gets even worse as we walk into the IVF clinic. I try to calm my nerves by telling myself that IVF is just a back-up plan. I have one more natural ovulation cycle before we start the IVF treatment. One more chance to make a baby as nature intended. Deep down, I know I'm kidding myself.

A bubbly, fresh-faced girl named Cindy directs us and three other couples into the conference room. I wonder if I should tell her about the ladder in her stocking. My anxiety quickly morphs into outrage when I discover that the 'girl' is actually the counsellor. At best, Cindy is in her mid-20s. It's possible she's even in her early 20s. Fresh out of university. Probably never even thought about making a baby. What does she know about fruitless conception sex and the heartbreak of infertility? Her knowledge could only be theoretical, in which case the IVF clinic could have just included another shiny brochure with the mail-order-baby catalogue and saved us all some time. And what is she so damn happy about?

I look around at the other couples and wonder which partner is broken. I diagnose the first couple as having old-man sperm. She's a 20-something Eastern European and he has got to be on his second or possibly third time around the marriage-go-round. The next couple are perfect-looking grown-up versions of figurines from the top of a wedding cake. Decked out in tailored pinstripes, he has a full head of hair with a distinguished peppering of grey. She's got glossy hair, a creamy complexion and a beautiful pink pashmina wrap. They both look to be in their mid to late 30s, so I guess either of them could be the dud. The third couple look young enough to still be fertile. They appear hippyish, you know, the type who'd own a VW Kombi van with a dolphin sticker on the window. I conclude that he must have smoked too much pot and damaged his little boys.

This may surprise you, but my rash and wholly unsubstantiated stereotypical generalisations turn out to be completely wrong, at least about the last couple. The hippy couple are both carriers of cystic fibrosis, so they are using IVF in order to screen their embryos. When both parents are carriers, there is a 25 per cent chance that the baby will be born with full-blown cystic fibrosis. We didn't discuss their recreational drug habits.

The other two couples don't disclose anything personal about themselves, and Chris and I don't either. When the work-experience stude . . . I mean Cindy, asks if I'd like to say something about myself I say no. She quickly moves on to how each of us is going to deal with the process emotionally. Apparently I'm going to cry a lot (check) and need to talk about it endlessly. Chris is going to retreat in silence to his caveman cave and play a lot of golf. Chris leans over to me and whispers, 'Does this mean I have to buy a set of clubs in order for it to work?'

With the non-niceties out of the way, we move on to the legal aspects of proceedings. Before we can start IVF, we need to agree as a couple what we will do with any leftover eggs, sperm or embryos if we break up, if either of us dies, if we both die or if we just don't want to use them. We can either donate them to research, donate to another couple or single person, or destroy them. Chris and I discuss and debate the options in the car on the way home and over the next few days. This is far more complex than I had ever imagined. We're forced to discuss the scenarios of life and death for both of us and our potential children, whether we donate our embryos to another couple or put them up for research.

One week later at the information session, we sit next to the wedding-cake-doll couple. Unlike last time, I decide to make an effort and introduce myself. Sharon is a lawyer and Murray is an estate agent. 'We both work such long hours we hardly see each other. That's the main reason we need IVF,' Sharon laughs. 'We don't have time to have sex.' It turns out that we live in the same neighbourhood, so Sharon and I agree to meet up at the weekend for a chat. She also gives me the name of her acupuncturist, who specialises in infertility and supporting IVF treatments.

The information night is truly terrifying. In fact, it could just as easily have been called 'Drugs That Should Never Have Been Approved For Use and That Really Ought to be Recalled Before Someone Gets

Hurt'. The nasal spray designed to stop your natural ovulation process, for example, has been known to induce suicidal thoughts, and the hormone injections are guaranteed to turn you into a moody bitch. And then there are the invasive internal scans and blood tests every two days, the risks of a general anaesthetic and surgery to collect the eggs, and the stirrup bed and metallic duck bill required for the embryo transfer.

At the end of it all, Chris leans over and whispers, 'If you were searching for evidence that God is a man, all you need do is come to an IVF information night. You get turned into a science experiment and all I have to do is wank into a cup.' The evening concludes with another reminder that women need to talk a lot throughout the process and men play a lot of golf. 'I knew there had to be a catch. Men don't get off so lightly after all,' Chris says. 'We're required to take up golf.'

# 20

# SHOOTING UP

We are sitting in the waiting room at the IVF clinic waiting for our lesson on how to shoot up. There are lots of needles and lots of injections involved in IVF, although this is something they don't put on the brochure with the price list. The reality of the situation is finally sinking in. We've been discussing my infertility and the potential of IVF for months, but I always felt like we were indulging in a game of 'what if?'. This was never going to happen to me. But yesterday when my period arrived and I flushed away my last chance of conceiving naturally, I could no longer deceive myself about my infertility.

I even started reading all the books I'd previously bought about IVF but thought I'd never need to read. They're horrible. I shouldn't be surprised. Any book that has a sun setting over a bland landscape with a rainbow on the front cover is almost certain to be about some horrible, bleak topic. They're also sickeningly earnest. Where are the gags? At a time like this I don't want to read about other people's sad stories. I want some light relief from the sense of failure that I'm unable to shake. I want to know that everything's going to be OK.

I look around the waiting room with the knowledge that I'll be here every 24 to 48 hours for God knows how long, a daily reminder that I am a sad, old, broken, infertile loser. Chris interrupts my wallowing by saying apologetically, 'I'm sorry, puss cat, but I'm so freaked out by needles I don't think I'll be able to give the injections to you.'

'That's OK,' I say stoically. 'I'll be able to do it myself.'

As soon as we walk into the nurse's office I can no longer maintain my stoic veneer. My eyes well with tears yet again. I bat them away and tell myself to be strong. They are just injections, after all, and I've had plenty of injections in my life. I don't cry when I get a tetanus injection, so why should I cry over this? The nurse sits us down in her office and explains our IVF protocol. Dr Lucy has decided that I'll skip the nasal spray that usually comes before the injections. I'm going straight for the jabs. The needles are in a thermal bag sitting on the nurse's desk. She unzips the bag to show us what's inside and prepares to demonstrate how to use them. 'Have you talked about who's going to give the injections?' she asks.

I burst into tears and start sobbing.

'I will,' says Chris.

The nurse demonstrates the injecting process with an orange. Then she clarifies that we won't actually inject an orange. Uh-huh. Check. Memo to self: don't try to medicate a citrus fruit. I'll have to grab a roll of fat on my stomach (finally! something I know without question that I can do) while Chris jabs the needle in.

At home, I phone Sharon so I can 'talk about it and express myself' as per the instructions at the information session. Sharon is a couple of weeks ahead of me in her protocol and has a whole week's experience of shooting up. She suggests I put ice on my belly before the injection. It numbs the area so it hurts less. It's also supposed to minimise the bruising. We use the ice trick that night when it's time for my first injection. I grab the roll of fat and Chris is about to inject me when I shout, 'Stop.' I can't watch him stab me, so I take the needle from him and do it myself. Toffee jumps off her pillow and runs over to me. She looks worried, ready to begin an intervention to prevent her human from starting a drug habit. Chris pats her and says, 'Don't worry, Toffee, this is hardly recreational.'

I don't know if it's the ice or my excellent needle technique, but I hardly feel a thing. 'I wonder how long it takes before I turn into a moody bitch?' I say.

'You'll be OK, puss cat,' Chris says.

The next morning is the day of Sharon's egg collection. I text her to wish her good luck. She texts straight back and says, 'It's 7 a.m. and I'm watching porn waiting for Murray to cum.'

How do I respond to that? 'I'm thinking of you' seems like the wrong thing to say, not least because I'm trying really hard not to think of Murray with his pants at his ankles watching a porno. I ask Chris what I should say and he suggests I text back, 'Well, you're in good hands. Estate agents are famous for being A-grade wankers.'

As soon as I walk into work, my boss comes over to my desk and tells me I've been assigned to a project with a financial institution. It's an initial six-month contract with a likely extension to twelve months. I start tomorrow. This financial institution also happens to be in another city. I will fly up there every week for up to a year. I hate travelling for work. I hate getting up early on Monday mornings to catch the red-eye flight and I hate eating plane food. Do you have any idea how many calories are in your standard in-flight meal? I don't mind consuming calories on good food and wine, but unidentified animal and shrivelled-up peas floating in a sea of fat are just not worth the calories. I also hate all the lonely nights in hotel rooms with only the mini-bar and pay TV for company. But I knew I'd have to travel when I took this job, so I'm in no position to back out now. The only sticking point is that my life has changed since then. I can't go anywhere any more because I have a date with the IVF clinic every day or two.

My boss reads the expression on my face and asks me what's wrong. I don't know what to tell him. Out of principle I don't want to discuss my infertility with him, so I decide to keep it vague. 'Due to personal reasons I'm not able to travel at the moment.'

'That's fine,' he says. 'Take this week to sort out whatever you have to and I'll arrange for you to start next week.'

'I can't travel next week either,' I say.

'Well, when can you travel?'

'I don't know,' I say.

I'm not deliberately being vague. I really don't know. Some people do IVF for years. In fact, my friend Cathy, who was on IVF for over two years, told me that the worst part of it, even worse than the emotional roller coaster and invasion of privacy, was having to put her life on hold. For years she was unable to plan anything. She and her husband couldn't go away on holidays or even arrange catch-ups with friends because of the constant rounds of scans, blood tests, acupuncture sessions, egg harvesting or egg transfers. I remember her telling me at the time that she had to do something every day. Even when she didn't have to go into the clinic, she still had to give herself an injection or take the nasal spray, and in most cases she was required to do it at an exact time every day too.

'You're going to have to give me more information,' my boss says.

In a split second, I assess my options. Do I lie and tell him I'm caring for a sick relative? Do I give him half the truth and tell him I'm undergoing urgent medical treatment? I can't bring myself to tell an outright lie and I also can't have him conclude that I have a serious health issue. I have no option but to tell the truth about my IVF treatment.

He suggests that I delay starting IVF until after the assignment, and I am forced to divulge even more private information that is none of my company's damn business. 'I can't delay for any length of time. This is my last chance of ever having a baby.'

As soon as I utter the 'b' word I know I've committed two corporate sins from which my career will never recover. The first is to let personal issues interfere with the job. By not taking this assignment, regardless of how valid the reason, I have shown that I do not have blind loyalty and unwavering commitment to the company. I am not worthy to sit at the hotdesk that has so generously been cleared so that I might temporarily sit at it. Worse than that – so much worse – I have admitted that I want to have a baby. The moment I said it, my boss probably calculated the loss of productivity due to placenta brain during pregnancy, the cost of paying for maternity leave and the inconvenience of an employee becoming an inflexible mother who is shackled by childcare pick-up times and the needs of her children. I know of women who desperately want children but, at work, constantly pretend that they don't. Now I know why they do it.

My boss accepts my reasons for refusing the assignment as gracefully as can be expected. He says he will smooth everything over with all the stakeholders but warns that it will not be looked on favourably, particularly when the time comes for discussing bonuses and pay rises. The outcome is bittersweet. I'm pleased that I don't have to travel for work, but I am also well aware that I have now been demoted to the mummy track. Motherhood is already denting my career prospects – and I'm not even pregnant and may never be.

If the situation had been reversed and Chris had been sent away for work, he would have been able to go. All he'd have to do is take a sick day on the day of the egg collection. He could fly home, have a wank and then fly back again. Sure, it's a long way to go to cum, but it wouldn't be the first time in history that a man has gone to extraordinary lengths to get his rocks off. I hate the injustice. I hate that regardless of laws and corporate policies, so long as women are the ones who have the babies, we will never be equal.

I once overheard a client say that he'll only employ a woman if he can't find a suitable man. Women are too much trouble, because eventually they all just go off and have babies. Even legislative changes mandating paid maternity leave have made things worse for women, not better, in terms of career progression. Comparative studies have shown that countries with the most generous family-friendly policies also have glass ceilings made from the thickest reinforced glass. Researcher Catherine Hakim writes in an article called 'The Mother of All Paradoxes', published in *Prospect Magazine*, that 'Onerous maternity protection leads the private sector to systematically avoid hiring women . . . The sad result is that the more generous the maternity rights, the less likely women are to reach the top.'

I stew all day over the toll that motherhood has already taken on my career. By the time I get home, I am furious. Chris walks into the apartment to see me banging doors, kicking cupboards and swearing like a trooper. I very rarely lose my temper, and I never lose it like this. I feel the rage of a lifetime of PMT concentrated into a single moment. It's almost like an out-of-body experience. I can see myself acting like a crazy lady, but I can't stop it. I'm completely out of control.

'Whatever I've done,' Chris says, 'I'm sorry.'

He delivers the line with his classic comic timing. I start to laugh, but it quickly morphs into sobbing. Chris holds me as I pummel his chest and cry it out. When I calm down, he says, 'Well, I guess the drugs are starting to kick in.'

# 21

## SPECIAL DELIVERY

I've turned into a pin cushion. Not only is my body full of pinpricks from the daily hormone injections and thrice-weekly acupuncture sessions, it has also become soft and squishy. I've put on two kilograms, and it's only been a few days. As I change into my blue hospital gown in preparation for yet another internal scan, I catch my reflection in the mirror. Is that cellulite on my belly or is it just a shadow? I remember my friend Cathy telling me that she put on fifteen kilograms during the two years or so she was undergoing IVF.

I've been poked and prodded so much in the last year that internal scans should be a walk in the park, but they don't get any easier. Spreading your legs for a complete stranger and having a cold metal object shoved up you is just not something that you get used to with practice. Today's scan is to check that my body is responding appropriately to the hormone injections. The hormones make your body produce more than one egg in a cycle. They're similar to the fertility drugs I was taking before, just on a much bigger scale. Instead of producing two or three eggs per cycle, this drug can make you produce as many as twenty eggs. Producing this many eggs is purely for efficiency. Because collecting the eggs involves a surgical procedure and because some of the eggs probably won't survive the collection or the fertilisation, the doctors like to have some spares on hand just in case. Any leftover embryos go in the deep freeze for next time.

People respond differently to the hormones, so Dr Lucy just makes an educated guess as to how much I should inject each day. If I inject too much, I could get what's called ovarian hyperstimulation, which is when your body releases too many eggs and you feel like you are going to split open and you end up in hospital from the potential risk of organ failure. Not enough hormones and your body will only release its normal one egg.

My new IVF pal Sharon had six eggs collected a couple of days earlier. She was so excited when she rang to tell me the news, only to ring back a few hours later with an update that only three of the six eggs had been fertilised. Then when her three little embryos were growing in their Petri dish, two of them kicked the bucket, which only left one embryo to transfer and none for the freezer. She was unable to disguise her disappointment when we caught up for yet another extra-large glass of vegetable juice. (Coffee is a luxury reserved for the fertile.)

'I bet they killed them deliberately,' Sharon says. 'They don't want more than one embryo to survive. They want you to have to go through another egg harvest so you pay all over again.'

I have to admit that Sharon has just hit on a great way for IVF clinics to improve their bottom line – particularly if they are fly-by-night operations who don't care a fig about medical ethics or their reputations. I resist pointing out to Sharon that people generally don't go into IVF to make a quick buck, and I decide against telling her that the idea that IVF clinics deliberately kill their clients' embryos is on the wrong side of crazy.

'How could all of them die except one?' Sharon continues. 'They could be lying to me and I wouldn't know.'

'Why would they lie to you?' I ask, sure that this is the drugs talking rather than the previously rational Sharon. 'If the embryos survived, what do you think they did with them?'

'They're probably selling them on eBay. I bet you can get a lot for an embryo online.'

I laugh awkwardly, because I'm only half sure that she's joking.

Sharon goes on to tell me about her friend who has been banned from doing any more cycles at the IVF clinic for 12 months because they are worried about her mental health. After her last failed cycle, she went into the clinic and said things like, 'I don't know why I'm bothering. I don't even know why you're bothering. I suppose you don't care. You're just taking my money and I'm just giving it to you.'

The IVF clinic should take some responsibility for this. Not once has the clinic volunteered information about their success rates. You don't have to dig too deeply to discover that on average it takes six or seven IVF cycles to conceive a baby. But you could very easily get the impression that you'll most likely conceive on your first cycle, or your second at the most. My acupuncturist tells me that if I can't afford to do at least four cycles, both financially and emotionally, then I should reconsider starting in the first place.

Back in the IVF clinic, I'm not surprised when the scan shows that only one of my ovaries is producing egg follicles. Dr Lucy was right. My fertility plane is now only flying on one engine – and even that isn't functioning at 100 per cent. Unfortunately, all of my egg follicles are much smaller than they should be. At this point, it's unclear if any of them will develop into anything worth harvesting.

The nurse tells me not to worry (yeah, right) and to come back tomorrow for yet another scan and blood test. In a way, I'm glad I've come clean with my boss about my IVF treatment. How else could I explain all these medical appointments?

The next day reveals no change. I'm given some extra injections, which are also extra big and extra expensive and leave extra big, extra expensive bruises. Two days later, I have another scan and things haven't improved. 'It's not looking good, is it?' I say to the nurse.

The nurse says it's not her place to comment on my progress. She doesn't have to. Her lack of eye contact says it all. I relay my concerns to Chris, and he optimistically suggests that the nurse may just have poor social skills.

I'm given yet another injection, so I'm now shooting up three times a day. Doing a quick calculation as to how much money I'm injecting into my body, I point out to Chris that a heroin habit would probably be cheaper. We laugh about it, but there's an underlying seriousness. The extra costs that weren't included in our original quote are mounting up. We've blown our budget by thousands of pounds, and it's only our first cycle. Chris tells me not to worry because everything will work out. After a phone call from Sharon, I dare to believe that he may be right. Sharon is pregnant! Ten agonisingly slow days after her embryo transfer, she has a blood test. Four even more agonisingly slow hours after that, the nurse phones to tell her she's pregnant. 'I can't believe it was this easy,' Sharon says. 'Lucky it worked first go, since I don't have any frozen embryos.'

The following week, my body has grown some eggs that are big enough to harvest. Now it's time for Chris to do his bit. Until we started IVF, I'd never really appreciated the pressure on the man to perform. I still think they get the easy part when you compare all the injections, blood tests and scans with just having to wank, but, nonetheless, cumming on demand and to the right specifications has its own pressures. There is a small window of time when the harvested egg must meet with the sperm. If the man is unable to provide the sperm on time, the egg will not be fertilised and the whole cycle will be wasted. After the physical and emotional turmoil of the past weeks, the idea of abandoning the cycle doesn't bear thinking about.

On the morning of my egg collection, I am a bundle of nerves. I try to conceal my anxiety from Chris because I don't want to put any more pressure on him than necessary. Failing miserably at disguising my anxiety, Chris orders me out of the bedroom while he gets down to business. Not long after, we are in the car on the way to the IVF clinic, with a vial of sperm tucked between my boobs to keep it warm.

We hand the precious vial over to the receptionist when we arrive at the clinic and then take a seat in the waiting room. What is the appropriate social etiquette for handing over a sperm sample to a stranger? Shyly handing it over with a whispered murmur seems unduly prudish, given that the whole reason we're here is to fertilise an egg. Then again, bounding up to the counter and declaring in a loud voice, 'Hi. Here's the sperm!' seems wrong. Luckily the hospital staff have developed their own social etiquette.

The room is filled with nervous-looking couples and women I presume to be single, many of whom look as if they've brought their mothers along. I estimate how much revenue the IVF clinic will be generating today and wonder if we are paying for someone's boat or house extension. There's a pile of pregnancy magazines on the table, which seems a little premature, not to mention insensitive. Could there be anything more inappropriate than shoving pictures of happy pregnant women in the faces of people who are about to have surgery to try to make a baby, knowing that for many it won't work?

A man wearing hospital greens goes to the counter and talks briefly with the receptionist. Both glance in our direction before the man approaches us. He seems more awkward and unsure than we do. He ushers us over to the other side of the room, presumably trying to create the illusion of privacy. If it is, it's a pretty piss-poor illusion, given that we're still in plain sight of everyone in the waiting room. Only now, everyone in the room is staring at us. And why wouldn't they? We look highly suspicious, huddling in the corner of an open-plan room. I feel like I'm taking part in a drug deal.

He introduces himself as the laboratory technician. 'I need to confirm your identity,' he whispers to Chris.

Chris whispers back his name, address and date of birth.

'Did you produce this sample yourself?' the technician whispers.

'Are you asking if I had help?' Chris asks with a mischievous look in his eye.

The man looks embarrassed. 'I . . . I . . . I mean,' he stutters, 'is this your sample? We need to check that it's your sperm and not somebody else's.'

Chris confirms that it's his, and the man from the lab nods and says thank you.

'You're welcome,' says Chris, no longer whispering, and with a big smile he says, 'The pleasure has been all mine! I've been practising for this day my whole life.'

Several more people ask if Chris produced his sperm sample on his own. Everyone is speaking in hushed and serious tones. It's doing my head in, and eventually I say to the nurse, 'Everyone around here seems a bit uptight.' The nurse laughs and says that working in the IVF clinic is like walking on eggshells. Patients regularly lose their tempers and direct their anger at the staff. She says that the men often struggle with having people handling and discussing their sperm and the women are so full of hormones you can't predict what they might do.

# 22

# EASTER BUNNY WEARS CROCS

**M**ore questions and more forms. Things are a blur until I find myself walking into the operating theatre, awkwardly holding my ugly blue surgical gown closed at the back. The operating theatre is cold and impersonal and full of medical staff. I try not to look at the surgical instruments laid out on the tray, instead focusing on the shoes of the doctors and nurses. I notice they are all wearing Crocs.

'Where's Dr Lucy?' I ask.

A masked man tells me that he'll be collecting my eggs today. 'Just call me the Easter Bunny,' he says.

He looks kind of young, too young for my liking. 'Have you done this before?' I ask.

'No, but I've taken out plenty of tonsils.'

That is the last thing I remember until I wake up in the recovery room to discover that they harvested six eggs.

'Well done, puss cat,' Chris says as he gives me a kiss. I'm ecstatic. I know that some, or even all, of them can die off between now and the transfer, but it seems like a miracle that I could make any eggs at all.

Later that day, as I'm resting at home, the nurse phones to tell me that one egg has died and the remaining five have been fertilised. 'But,' she cautions, 'it's too early to get excited.' Dr Lucy has instructed that my embryos are to be grown to blastocysts. Typically the embryos

159

are grown in the Petri dish for two days until they have multiplied into four cells. Because my egg quality is poor, the lab will grow them for five days until they have multiplied into blastocysts, which comprise many cells. The reason for this is that the crappy ones will die during the five days and the ones that survive to become blastocysts will be the strongest and will have the best chance of making a baby. There's no point transferring a crappy embryo after two days if it's going to die anyway.

This method, however, is not without risks. First, all the embryos may die and there will be none to transfer. And second, embryos grown to blastocysts before they are transferred are six times more likely to split into identical twins. At this point, I'm not thinking about the risk of twins. All I want is for one of our little fellas to survive the next five days.

Five days later, we arrive at the IVF clinic and discover that four of them have made it. Unlike the egg collection, Chris is allowed into the operating theatre with me for the transfer. I guess this is the closest we're going to get to 'conceiving' our child, so it's good of them to let Chris be present. We are shown a magnified photo of our embryo. It looks like a turtle – the most beautiful turtle I've ever seen. I start to cry as I realise that I'm looking at a picture of my baby.

The nurse asks if my bladder is full. Oh shit. I went to the toilet about ten minutes before, when I changed into my hospital gown. I knew I wasn't supposed to wee. They told us at the briefing session, and then again when they phoned to confirm the time of my procedure. But I forgot. I always need to pee when I'm nervous and anxious.

The doctor comments on my empty bladder when I'm lying on the table. 'We like a full bladder because it makes it easier to see where to put the embryo.'

I panic. Have I ruined everything? 'You're not going to put it in the wrong place, are you?' I ask. 'You won't put it in my bladder by mistake?'

The doctor laughs at me and so does the nurse. 'Your body doesn't work that way. It's a completely different hole.'

I relax a bit more after his reassurance that he will still be able to put the embryo in the right place, but I can't help but feel guilty. I feel like I've failed the test of motherhood at the very first hurdle. I had one simple instruction and I cocked it up. Is this mother-guilt starting already?

Chris holds my hand as a strange man who I've never met before and am unlikely to ever meet again impregnates me with a long tube containing my darling little turtle.

'Are you sure it is my embryo you just shoved up there?' I ask.

The doctor looks confused, so I clarify. 'Are you sure it's my embryo and not somebody else's?' Ever since I started the IVF process, I've had a recurring nightmare that my egg or Chris's sperm will get mixed up in the IVF lab. I worry that our baby will come out with ethnic features different from ours. Everyone will know that it can't possibly be ours and we'll have to give it back.

The doctor reassures me. 'We have very strict procedures on these things.'

I decide to give him the benefit of the doubt, but something else is worrying me too. 'How will I know if the embryo falls out?' I ask.

'It won't fall out,' the doctor laughs. 'Think of it like a strawberry seed in a jam sandwich. You can turn the sandwich upside down and shake it, but the seed won't move because it's wedged between two pieces of bread.'

As I'm changing out of the gown and back into my clothes I feel a surge of emotion, so I ask Chris to pull the curtain around my cubicle. As soon as it's closed I start to sob, gut-wrenching sobs. I don't know why I'm crying. I should be happy. I have a little turtle in a jam sandwich and three leftover embryos in the freezer. Maybe I am happy, maybe I'm sad, maybe I'm scared and maybe I'm excited. Chris hugs me until my tears subside, then he says that he ought to smoke a cigar and swill some whisky, since we've just conceived a child. We settle for yet another vegetable juice instead.

# 23

# PLANT A FUCKING TREE

Now it's my turn to endure the ten-day wait. I was warned in the briefing session that this would feel like the longest ten days of my life. They weren't kidding. It isn't just me that is finding it hard. If Chris owned golf clubs, or didn't think that golf is possibly the dullest game in the world, he may well have disappeared to the green by now. Instead he spends every spare moment sitting on his computer teaching himself a computer programming language. I question him on his new interest in cutting code and he says, 'Computer programming language makes sense. I know that if I do certain things I'll get a predictable result. It's like escaping into a world of pure, crystalline logic. It feels like the only thing with any certainty at the moment.'

On day two, Sharon phones with horrible news. Her baby has died. She had a scan a couple of days earlier to check for a heartbeat and discovered that her baby was smaller than it should be. It was only one millimetre smaller, but apparently that's a big deal at this stage in the pregnancy. Dr Lucy warned Sharon that it didn't look good. Sharon returned for another scan today and discovered that there was no longer a heartbeat. 'I have a dead baby inside me,' she sobs into the phone. 'I have to carry a dead baby around inside me until I miscarry.'

I don't know what to say. What is there to say? At times like this, our language fails us. I tell her that I'm so sorry and am instantly struck by how pathetic a response it sounds, but what else is there? When she visits Cindy the perky IVF counsellor for help dealing with her grief, Cindy suggests she writes a poem or plants a tree.

Plant a fucking tree? Another grossly inadequate response. Cindy also tells her that she needs to think about why she wants a baby so desperately. She sees a lot of women who are clinging to the hope of having a baby to fix their life or their marriage, or to give up work. 'It puts so much pressure on each cycle and also on the child,' Cindy says. 'A child won't fix your life. You need to fix your life first before you are ready to take on a baby.'

Again, I'm not sure this is the best advice for Sharon at a time like this.

Just like my friend Danielle's grief for her infertility after her attempts at IVF failed, miscarriage is another example of where there is no social ritual to help people grieve and cope. It's a silent and lonely grief. Most people don't even know that you've made a person, and even if they do, they often don't think about miscarriage as a death. Before I started IVF, before I saw my little turtle, an embryo was just a collection of cells. I put it in the same category as a bit of saliva or a piece of hair. I didn't think about an embryo as a life. But now I do. Even though my little turtle is barely more than the size of a pinhead, it's already a person. It's my baby.

And now Sharon's baby is dead, and all we can offer her are empty words and stupid gardening advice.

# 24

# VINEGAR AND PARMESAN

'I want some vinegar,' I say to Chris four days after the transfer. Sharon's heartbreak is still weighing heavily on my mind. Usually when I'm sad I want chocolate, but today my comfort food of choice is vinegar.

'Do you want some salt and vinegar crisps?' Chris clarifies.

'Not that sort of vinegar,' I say, making a beeline for a health-food shop, leaving Chris in my wake. I want apple cider vinegar. Before it's paid for, I unscrew the lid and take a swig. Chris and the shop assistant stare at me. 'I can't tell you how good this tastes,' I say as I take another swig. 'Do you think this means I'm pregnant?' I ask hopefully.

'They said it's too early to tell, puss cat,' Chris says.

That night, I wake up at 2 a.m. with a hunger that can only be cured by cheese. At 2.05 a.m., there are two cheese slices, half a block of cheddar and some grated Parmesan in the fridge. By 2.10 a.m., I've transferred all of it to my belly.

I wake Chris and ask, 'Do you think this means I'm pregnant?'

'They said it's too early to tell, puss cat,' Chris says. 'Go back to sleep.'

On day six after my transfer, my cheese craving returns. I'm at work, so I run to the grocery store and buy a large block of Parmesan. It can't be just any Parmesan. All of them except one particular brand smell so bad they make me want to vomit. Sitting at my desk munching on the block of cheese, trying not to attract attention to myself, I ring Chris, and guess what he says? 'They said it's too early to tell, puss cat.'

The suspense is killing me. I give in and buy a pregnancy test. We have been warned so many times by the IVF clinic that I shouldn't do a home pregnancy test. The drugs I took just before the egg collection can cause a false positive pregnancy-test result. It's highly likely that the result will just create false hope that will only be dashed a few days later by the blood-test results. But I can't help it. I have to know.

I wee on the stick and then three minutes later I wish I hadn't. Negative. My heart sinks. I feel so foolish. How stupid of me to think that it would work. I'm infertile, I'm barren, I have rubbish eggs. As if I could make a baby. I don't tell Chris about the test. I'm too upset and too embarrassed.

I worry depression is setting in, because the next morning I can't get out of bed. I'm so tired, as if I could sleep for a hundred years and it still wouldn't be enough. Dragging myself into the shower, I feel too exhausted to stand, so I turn around and crawl back into bed. But I can't sleep, because I have to keep getting up to wee.

On the ninth day I'm still exhausted, but I'm quite sure I'm not depressed. I don't feel even a little bit down. Against my better judgement – and that of the entire medical profession – I buy another pregnancy test and can't believe my eyes when the magical second line appears as soon as I start weeing on the stick. I call Chris in excitement only to wonder part way through our conversation if the test is faulty. 'It's supposed to take three minutes for the positive line to appear,' I say. 'It took less than three seconds; do you think that means that test isn't valid?'

Chris has the patience of a saint, but I know I've pushed it too far when he says, 'Kasey, will you just wait until the blood test? It's only one more sleep.'

Actually, it's more accurate to say that it is one more night, because I certainly can't get any sleep.

As I'm sitting in the waiting room of the IVF clinic, I'm hoping that it's the last time I have to come here. I hate this place. I've spent so much time here over the last couple of months, but I'm still not used to it. I still have to choke back tears every time I walk through the door.

I confess to the nurse taking my blood that I did a pregnancy test yesterday. She shakes her head and says, 'We have very clear guidelines about that.'

'I know, but I couldn't help it,' I say.

'I understand completely,' she says. 'People think we don't understand what you're going through, that we don't care. But we do.'

She wishes me luck and says somebody will phone me in four hours with the results. I go straight to work, but I can't concentrate. In fact, I can't even sit still. It's like I've contracted ADHD. I can't bear to be around people, so I tell the receptionist that I'll be working from home for the rest of the day. Of course, I don't do any work except for one phone call that I can't avoid. I dial in for a phone conference with some colleagues and make the requisite 'aha' noises when appropriate. As if I could care about change management at a time like this. Chris is at home too and is struggling with similar concentration issues. When a call comes through on the other line, I hang up on my colleagues without any warning and take the other call.

It's the IVF clinic. The nurse says, 'I'm ringing with your test results.' And then she pauses for a cruel and unnecessarily long period of time – or at least that's how it seems. I feel like I'm on a game show and the host is about to tell me if I've won a million dollars . . . right after the commercial break. Chris is standing at the door, watching me at a distance. I can't read his expression. The commercial break ends and the nurse says, 'You're pregnant.'

I've fantasised about receiving this phone call a hundred times. Each time I imagined myself behaving as if I were indeed on a game show. I would squeal with delight and burst into tears and Chris would run down from the audience and embrace me. But the reality is quite different. All I can say is, 'Oh, right. Well, thanks for letting me know.' I hang up the phone and Chris is still standing at the door with a blank expression on his face.

'Well?' he says.

After a time, I say, 'Oh my God, we're going to have a child.'

Chris doesn't squeal with delight either. He wraps his arms around me and we're silent for a long time. I know how ridiculous this sounds, but I've been so focused on getting pregnant it has been ages since I've thought about babies and motherhood.

'Nobody told us that having a baby was a side effect of IVF!' Chris quips with mock outrage.

'I'm going to be a mum and you're going to be a dad,' I say as the tears begin to flood into my eyes.

'Well done, puss cat. We did it.'

# 25

# NO PAIN, NO GAIN

'Will you accept children lovingly into your lives?' the priest asks as he stands at the altar of the tiny sandstone church.

'I will,' I reply. But it would be more accurate to say 'I have.' One month after the phone call that changed our lives, I'm a pregnant bride. I'm obviously not waddling down the aisle with a bulging belly, but I do need emergency alterations to the top of my wedding dress. My boobs are enormous. Already! And they were huge from the fertility drugs anyway.

Initially I decided to get married for the good of my baby and because it was important to Chris. I didn't expect marriage to have any impact at all on me or on my relationship with Chris. I love Chris and I am committed to him. I couldn't see how a ceremony and a piece of paper could add anything more.

But it does. I now have a sense of security that I never knew existed and didn't know I was missing. I know that almost half of all marriages break up. (It's hard to escape this fact when bitter, or perhaps wise, divorcees say things like, 'Don't change your name, love, it's too hard to change it back.') Nonetheless, I'm enjoying the security and optimism that comes from making a public commitment to each other. I wonder how long it will be before I stop giggling when I say 'my husband' and stop cringing when Chris says 'my wife'.

While I am both delighted and terrified to be pregnant, I'd be lying

169

if I tell you I'm enjoying it. I struggle through the first three months with a sense of hope. All the pregnancy books talk about how wonderful the second trimester is, with the glowing skin, thick silky hair and all the happy hormones coursing through a pregnant body. A friend tells me that when she was pregnant she was so horny she had orgasms in her sleep. Now that's something I wouldn't mind trying. But the second trimester comes and goes, and I do not. Well, not in my sleep. I'm now seven months in and there hasn't been the slightest hint of getting hot under the collar in my dreams. In fact, I've never felt more unsexy in my life. I have had constant nausea, I'm uncomfortable all the time, and call me crazy, but spontaneously peeing my pants just doesn't do it for me.

You'd think that morning sickness would have made me stick-thin with just a cute little baby bump out the front. But it hasn't. Eating is the only thing that gives me any relief from nausea. So I eat day and night, and I've already gained over 20 kg. I am so fat that when I lie in bed I feel like an upturned beetle. I can't sit up, so I have to rock back and forth to get some momentum so I can roll out of bed. My lowest point comes at eight months, when I realise that my legs and hips touch the sides of the bath. I'm so worried that I'll get stuck in the bath that I only have one when Chris is home, in case I need rescuing.

To make matters worse, it seems that every time I leave the house somebody feels the urgent need to mention my weight gain, as if, somehow and inexplicably, it has escaped my notice. Even the woman who comes to our apartment to measure up the curtains for the nursery gives me unsolicited advice. 'Oh, honey, I see you've put weight on your hips and bum,' she says. 'I hate to tell you this, but it's not true what they say. The weight doesn't come off with breastfeeding. It's even worse if it's an IVF baby. Yours isn't an IVF baby, is it?' When I nod, she says, 'Oh well, then you'll never get rid of it.'

Some people are 'kinder' and tell me that I am carrying my baby weight really well and I'm lucky not to have a fat face. Regardless of whether they are being kind or cruel, it bothers me that we are talking about it at all. When everyone else is so obsessed with my weight gain, whether it be too much, too little (I don't think anybody has ever said that to me) or just enough, I can't help but get fixated on it myself. I know I shouldn't worry about it. I'm pregnant, for fuck's sake, and I'm carrying a healthy baby. Surely that's all that matters. There are more important things to worry about than whether or not I'm getting a puffy face.

But then I come across health professionals who seem to be no better than the curtain lady. In the waiting room of Dr Olivia, my obstetrician, I flick through a book on pregnancy written by a male doctor suggesting that pregnant women plot a graph of their weekly weight gain compared with the recommended weight gain. They can create a baseline by noting their pre-conception weight and then adding on the 'normal' weight gain for each week or month. The doctor suggests that by weighing themselves every week, women can plot with scientific accuracy exactly how big a failure they have become over the course of their pregnancy, thereby creating the optimum growing conditions for a dose of the baby blues – even before the bub has arrived. OK, so I made that last bit up. But he might as well have written that.

The doctor also says that it's a shame there is an emerging trend amongst obstetricians not to weigh their patients at every visit. No doubt this same doctor hankers for a time when high-waisted bell-bottomed trousers were fashionable, ABBA wasn't considered nostalgic and *Are You Being Served?* was considered funny. In the 1970s, my mum's doctor weighed her at every visit when she was pregnant. Mum said that her doctor used to make her feel so bad about gaining too much weight that she would starve herself the day before her appointment. The day of the appointment she would still be reprimanded for putting on too much weight. Then for days after the appointment she would feel guilty about depriving her babies of nutrients.

Susan Maushart claims in *The Mask of Motherhood* that women can't win when it comes to pregnancy weight. Maushart quotes a study of body-image experiences among 63 pregnant women that found that pregnant women felt anxious about their weight gain regardless of how little or how much they actually gained. 'Clearly, we are deeply invested with the notion that there is a "correct" way for our bodies to perform pregnancy – and that everyone else is achieving the standard except ourselves,' she writes. 'That we should be conforming to someone else's standard is bad enough. But that we should be struggling so hard to conform to no one else's standard is truly remarkable.'

I ask Dr Olivia why she doesn't weigh me at my appointments. 'I'm sure you don't need me to tell you when you hit 80 kg,' she replies, adding that she can tell by looking at me that my weight gain is fine. Despite her reassurances, I stupidly volunteer to stand on her scales. What am I thinking? We discover that my weight gain is indeed above average. A few minutes earlier, Dr Olivia had scanned my baby and told me that it was below average in size. There is only one conclusion to draw: if my weight gain is above average and my baby's weight is below average, and people are telling me that I haven't put on weight in my face, then clearly all the fat has gone to my arse. No wonder my maternity clothes are getting tight. I recently discovered a design flaw in maternity clothes. They only put the elastic or the stretchy bit around the belly. But it isn't just my belly that has expanded. My back is enormous, and my cup size would have Pamela Anderson feeling inadequate. As for my hips and bum? The curtain lady did actually have a point.

I relay my concerns about my weight to my brother Wesley, who is a doctor. Wesley gives me the sweetest answer possible. He says that women put on the amount of weight that they need. If you're little to start with then you're going to put on more weight. He says that the reason my weight gain is above average is because the average woman is heavier than me to start with, so she doesn't need to gain as much weight. I don't think this theory accounts for all the weight I've gained. At eight and a half months, I foolishly weigh myself again and discover that I'm getting dangerously close to a 30-kg increase. And I was hardly a waif to start with. Nevertheless, Wesley's theory certainly makes me feel a little better.

Chris doesn't care about my weight gain either. I ask him one night if he can love a woman with cankles. He says, 'I've been loving her for a few weeks now.'

'I've had cankles for a few weeks?' I ask in horror. 'Why didn't you tell me?'

'I didn't think you needed to know,' he replies.

It is the same when I discover my stretch marks. We don't have a full-length mirror at home, so I haven't noticed them because they are low down on my belly, on the underside of my bump. It isn't until we are staying in a hotel that I discover them in the floor-to-ceiling mirror. 'Why didn't you tell me?' I demand.

'I didn't think you needed to know,' Chris says again, grinning mischievously.

I am truly amazed and baffled at his ability to find anything sexy. His theory is that men have a much greater range of what's sexy than they're often credited for. Sometimes this leads to Weirdsville, such as men who get off on wearing a nappy and being changed by women. On the upside, though, and for the most part, it means that men are capable of finding all kinds of women sexy, no matter what their shape or look.

Chris says that sleeping with a pregnant woman is like sleeping with a different woman every night, because my body is changing so much. It occurs to me that if Chris finds me sexy when I am close to 30 kg heavier than usual, have cellulite on my knees and stretch marks so bad I look like a sunburned zebra, then why did I used to worry and feel unsexy when my weight would fluctuate by a mere couple of kilograms? I could have saved myself so much self-condemnation and insecurity. Not for the last time, I wonder why we set such impossibly high standards for ourselves and then beat ourselves up when inevitably we can't meet them.

We recently discovered that our darling little turtle has grown into a darling little girl. It makes me wonder if my hang-ups about body image and perfection will be transferred to our daughter, or if in trying to avoid these hang-ups I will simply contribute to creating a whole new set just for her. Chris and I have been discussing baby names almost every day since we discovered the gender. We can't agree. He likes Polly and I want to name her Violet. I feel unqualified to pick a name for somebody, especially when I don't know what she's going to be like or what she'll want out of life. So we agree that whatever we choose, it must be a name that won't limit her opportunities. She needs a name that will enable her to be prime minister or a stripper or anything in between.

# 26

# PREGNANCY IS A COMPETITIVE SPORT

If somebody has to remind you to enjoy yourself then it's highly likely that whatever you're doing isn't inherently enjoyable. Nobody has ever had to instruct me to enjoy myself when I go out with friends, read a good book, eat a block of chocolate or have an orgasm. I enjoy them because they're enjoyable. For me, pregnancy is not. Yet I am constantly amazed by all the earth-mother types who tell me that I should be making the most of my pregnancy and enjoying it.

Pregnancy has not lived up to the oft-repeated claims that it is a spiritual experience either. I haven't had heightened spiritual awareness and so far I've been unable to tap into a 'powerful inner knowingness', as one website claims I should. The only thing I have worshipped for the last eight and a half months is the toilet bowl. When I tell my friend Brandy that I shouldn't complain about the nausea because I'm so lucky to be pregnant, she reminds me that my nausea started with the drugs I took to improve my egg quality, long before I was even pregnant. 'Complain all you want, babe,' she says. 'You've been throwing up for over a year.'

I have spent the entire pregnancy terrified of childbirth, until now. Now I am so uncomfortable I will gladly put up with anything just to get the baby out. Again, I am constantly bombarded by unwelcome and unhelpful comments about childbirth. A complete stranger says to me at a party, 'Are you worried about giving birth?'

Of course I am, but I hardly want to discuss it with him. I lie and say, 'No.'

'Well, you should be,' he replies like a precocious schoolboy intent on showing off his superior knowledge in front of an adult. 'Do you have any idea how many things could go wrong? You could die, you know.'

Who is this guy? And at what point did he decide that it might be a good idea to model his personality on C3PO? It's quite obvious by looking at me that childbirth is a couple of weeks, if not days, away. I am powerless to do anything to prevent childbirth and, if my new cyborg friend is to be believed, my impending death. Pity the poor woman who has C3PO's hand to hold while she's going through labour.

It isn't just dying that worries me. I'm terrified of the pain. A comedian I heard a few years ago put it best when she said, 'I don't even want to do something that feels good for 40 hours.' The constant pressure to have a drug-free birth doesn't help either. At the hospital birthing classes, it all appears very open-minded on the surface. The midwives say things like, 'Do what's best for you and for your baby. You can have as much or as little pain relief as you like.' But then a woman who gave birth the day prior comes in and speaks to the class. She tells us about her birthing experience, and the midwife prods her to tell us how long the labour lasted and what pain relief she used. When the new mother says she didn't use any pain relief, the midwife congratulates her.

Why is she being congratulated for having a drug-free birth when we were just told it doesn't matter? Despite the non-judgemental, open-minded rhetoric we've been given for the previous three hours, the clear and implicit message of the class is that it is better, or more womanly, or more moral, to do it without pain relief. I wonder what would have happened if the woman had said she had used drugs? Would the midwife be so positive? Or would she quickly move proceedings on to fun subjects like stitches and residual bladder leakage?

A few days later, I bump into the same midwife from the birthing class in a cafe. In her civvies she no longer feels like she needs to toe the hospital's inclusive line: that we should do what's right for us. She tells me that I should do everything I can to avoid having an epidural. She says that studies have shown that sheep that have epidurals don't bond with their young.

When I relay her advice to Chris, he says, 'Sheep!? She is aware that we're planning a human birth and not popping out Shaun the Sheep, isn't she? Had she looked at any studies that included people?'

Throughout my pregnancy, Chris has been amazed that pregnancy seems to be a competitive sport. Women compete about weight gain, how much we sacrifice our diets and lifestyles and, of course, how much pain we can endure at childbirth. But this midwife has just taken things to a new level. 'Not only do you have to compete with other women,' Chris says, 'now you have to compete with livestock as well.'

In the lead-up to the birth, I hear more stories about Evil Women Who Take Drugs During Birth. A friend of Emma's was induced and decided to have an epidural at the same time. Her labour lasted for six hours, during which she sat on the bed with her husband, playing cards and eating her favourite chocolates until it was time to push. Since then, she has been bombarded with questions about the birth. Everyone wants to know whether or not she had an epidural and how long she lasted before she succumbed. When she tells them she had one straight away, she gets raised eyebrows or judgemental looks, as if she is weak or has somehow failed. The health of her baby seems to come a distant second to her willingness to avail herself of the benefits of medicine. Her mother-in-law felt the need to remind her that she delivered all of her children without any pain relief at all.

Around the same time, Dr Denis Walsh, associate professor in midwifery at Nottingham University, provokes a storm of controversy by saying that women should avoid epidurals because they need to experience the pain of childbirth to prepare them for motherhood. Dr Walsh claims that 'Pain in labour is a purposeful, useful thing which has a number of benefits, such as preparing a mother for the responsibility of nurturing a newborn baby.' The mind boggles at this, even more so because the midwife in question is a man. Unless medical science takes a quantum leap in the next few years, he will never experience childbirth – or the pain of childbirth. His contribution to the debate on epidurals is like the opinion of the aristocrat from central casting who thinks that hunger and grinding poverty are necessary evils since they're the only things that can spur the indolent to work. By claiming that women need to feel the pain to be good mothers, is he also suggesting that women who have epidurals or C-sections are not good mothers? And if women need to experience pain to prepare themselves for motherhood, surely men ought to need a similar dose of pain to prepare themselves for fatherhood. Fathers need to bond with their children too. What about those women who are lucky enough to have quick labours and manageable pain? Does this mean that they are inferior to those who have a 40-hour labour with a baby in a posterior position?

I ask Dr Olivia if a drug-free birth is superior in any way. When she says 'no', I ask why people don't get an epidural at the first contraction and spare themselves all the pain.

'I have no idea,' she says.

'Is it bad for the baby if I have an epidural early in the labour?' I clarify.

'No.'

'So why do people endure hours of pain when they don't have to?'

Dr Olivia shrugs and says, 'Some people consider the pain of childbirth to be an opportunity for personal growth. My advice is to experience three contractions so you know what it feels like, then go straight for the epidural if you want it.'

When I relay this advice to a friend, she says that 'Childbirth is a really beautiful and natural experience. If you're bullied by the doctors into having drugs and medicalising the experience then you'll regret it.' This friend is childless.

And it doesn't stop at drugs. No sir! People have strong opinions about every minute detail of the birthing process, and they will let you know where you have erred for free and without prompting. If you should dare to have a different view about your own birth – or, worse, don't care one way or the other – they will denounce you just as quickly as if you suggested drowning kittens is not only fun but also a noble act.

Take birth plans, for instance. When I tell people that I don't have one, they look at me as if I am irresponsible and negligent. I don't have a birth plan, not because I haven't given the birth any thought – believe me, it is constantly on my mind – but because I haven't the slightest idea of what to put in it. Having never given birth before, I don't know how I am going to feel and what I am going to want. Sure, I've read lots of books about other women's experiences of giving birth, but buying a couple of squishy balls to help with the pain and learning some simple breathing exercises surely doesn't require a plan. A birth plan seems like setting myself up for failure. As my brother Wesley says, 'Babies have their own birth plans and have a remarkable disrespect for whatever their mother has written.' (Chris insists that we do have a birth plan. He calls it the Bruce Lee Birth Plan, after the kung fu expert. 'We have developed an approach to birth with no fixed positions,' Chris says. 'We'll be like water.')

And then there is where you decide to give birth. I meet an equally heavily pregnant woman at a party and she tells me she's planning a home birth because if she is in a hospital she'll probably be tempted to use drugs. 'What's wrong with that?' I ask. She replies, 'My husband wants me to have a natural, drug-free birth.' If a woman wants to have a drug-free birth, then good on her. All power to you, sista. But doing so because your husband expects it appals me. I just can't understand how a husband could possibly think he is entitled to dictate what his wife can and can't do with her body – especially when it comes to the sensation of pain, which is necessarily private: no one else can feel your pain. What sort of man would pressure his wife to go through excruciating pain if she didn't have to – or want to? Surely childbirth is hard enough without having the added pressure that you might disappoint your husband. While many of the criticisms of drugs in childbirth seem to be underpinned by a concern that birth has been medicalised – and therefore controlled by men – it seems that some of these women taking alternative approaches are no better off. They are still doing things in an attempt to please men.

But maybe I'm the weird one. It seems everywhere I turn I hear stories of women having their birth dictated to them by men. In the last couple of weeks I've become obsessed with watching birthing documentaries on pay TV, which seems to have whole channels devoted to playing birth documentaries around the clock. One show featured a woman who'd been in labour for twenty-one hours and was only one centimetre dilated. She was in agony and clearly distraught. She wanted an epidural, but her husband said no. He said that she wasn't a quitter and that she needed to be strong.

After enduring another four hours, she was only three centimetres dilated. At this point, hysteria set in. She said she couldn't do it any more. It had been 25 hours and her labour was just getting started. She begged her husband to let her get an epidural and, reluctantly, he agreed. He went outside to the waiting room to tell his mother, aunt and sisters the terrible news that his wife had had an epidural. What business was it of theirs or anyone's what pain relief his wife used? All the female members of the family looked disappointed.

In a follow-up interview, the husband said that he was disappointed that his wife 'gave in' and had an epidural. I don't even know the woman, but if I had been at the birth I would have wanted to do anything I could to help her. How could this guy watch somebody he loved in so much pain for so many hours and not want her pain to be alleviated?

The idea that one method of birth is superior to another is absurd to me. I've always viewed childbirth as purely a means to an end. It's all about getting the baby from the inside to the outside. The process of how that happens is of no consequence to me at all. The only things that I really care about are the health of my baby and my own health. I don't feel like I need to use childbirth to prove my womanhood, my self-worth, my pain tolerance or anything else. Which is just as well, because as it turns out my baby's birth is not an opportunity to prove any of these things.

# 27

# YAY! FOR THE EPIDURAL

Warning: I'm about to detail my birth experience. Some people love hearing about birthing stories and other people hate it. If you fall into the latter group then you'll probably want to skip this chapter.

One week after my due date, both my blood pressure and my baby are riding high. My baby hasn't 'dropped' into the birthing position, so I am seeing Dr Olivia for daily check-ups. By 'check-up' I mean she sticks her whole hand up me and pokes my cervix. She's worried that my blood pressure is too high. This is hardly surprising. Her blood pressure would go sky-high too if somebody subjected her to these 'check-ups' on a regular basis. But she doesn't want to take any risks, so she decides to induce me.

As Dr Olivia is applying the gel to 'marinate my cervix' and hopefully induce labour, I am still wondering if I've done the right thing. Do I really want to be a mother? Will I be any good at it? The gel is supposed to take 12 to 24 hours to work, so the plan is that Chris and I will go home for our last night as a childless couple and then come back in the morning. But about two minutes after the gel is applied, I start feeling pains. The midwife assisting Dr Olivia assures me that the pains aren't contractions because the gel doesn't work that fast. But because I am experiencing 'discomfort' (her choice of words, not mine), I am told to stay overnight. So much for enjoying our last night of childless freedom together. Chris is sent home and I am given a sleeping tablet. 'A sleeping tablet?' I ask hopefully. 'Does this mean I could sleep through the labour bit?' The midwife shakes her head and smirks at my ignorance. 'So it's unlikely I'll wake up in the morning and there will be a baby in the bed?' I say.

I tell her again that my 'discomfort' is really hurting, and she assures me again that it isn't labour. This frightens the hell out of me, because the pain is already excruciating. If this isn't labour, I don't know how I will cope when it does start. Unable to sleep, I start pacing around the room. Smacking my stress balls together, I repeat the mantra, 'It won't last, it won't last.' And a little voice inside is mocking me, saying, 'Are you serious? It hasn't even started yet.' About half an hour later, I am sitting on the toilet (for some reason this makes me feel better) and I hear a pop and then a gush of water. I'm not sure if I've peed without knowing (which has happened quite a lot over the last few weeks) or if my waters have broken. Looking into the toilet, I am pretty sure it's my waters. Whatever it is in the toilet, it isn't wee. It is a murky pink colour and reminds me of a petrol slick. As I stare into the toilet, the pain noticeably increases. Surely this is labour now. I call the midwife, but when she looks into the toilet bowl she says, 'I'm not convinced.'

'What do you mean you're not convinced?' I say, a little too forcefully. 'If that's not my waters then what is it?'

'I don't know,' she says, and instructs me to go back to bed. I do as I'm told, but on my way back to bed more of the murky fluid gushes out. Suddenly the midwife is a believer. She tells me to call Chris to tell him to come back to the hospital. 'Tell him not to rush,' the midwife instructs. 'It'll be hours before the labour really starts going.' I relay the 'don't rush' message to Chris and regret it as soon as I hang up. I don't care if I'm not in labour. It fucking hurts and I don't want to be here alone. The midwife puts a monitor on my belly and says with surprise, 'Oh, you are in labour. Your contractions are two minutes apart. That's unusual, the gel's not supposed to work that fast.'

By the time Chris arrives, I am delirious with pain. 'The stress balls are fucking useless,' I snap at him by way of greeting. The only thing I can do is hold Chris's hands and count through the contractions. After about seven hours and almost no progress, the midwife asks if I'd like an epidural. I had been so caught up in the pain I'd completely forgotten about the possibility of pain relief. *Hooray!* for medical science. I *love* my epidural. After it kicks in, I relax back on the bed and Chris curls up on the chair. He goes to sleep, but I can't. I'm exhausted, but I can't relax enough to sleep. Being poked and prodded every 20 minutes by a midwife doesn't help my chances of sleep much either.

Six hours later, Dr Olivia and a midwife are poking and prodding me when all of a sudden the machines start beeping and the medical professionals go quiet. Another midwife rushes in and the three of them stand together talking in hushed tones. Something is wrong. Chris and I exchange a worried glance. At this moment, I know how sheer terror feels. A couple of minutes pass, which feel like an eternity, and Dr Olivia announces that I'm going in for an emergency C-section. My baby is stuck in my pelvis and her heart rate is unstable. I don't know if it is my panic or just the exhaustion, but as soon as I am wheeled into the operating theatre I vomit.

Chris sits beside me, holding my hand. 'I really hope she's not Asian or black,' I say. The nurses look at me awkwardly, probably thinking I am racist, a slut or perhaps both. I don't have the energy to explain my IVF mix-up fears, although, at this point, they're the least of my worries. I just want her to be OK.

I feel a pull and hear a little cry. It's the sweetest sound I've ever heard. My baby is on the outside and she's alive. Little Violet Polly is lifted above the screen. I want to say that I am consumed by a feeling of love, but I'm not. My only feeling is one of nausea. While Violet is being cleaned up and checked out I am given some anti-nausea medication, so when she is brought to me I am at least able to recognise that I am looking at my baby and start to register the magnitude of the occasion.

The next days are a blur of sleeplessness and trying to get the hang of breastfeeding. On day three, the baby blues kick in, right on schedule. I know they've arrived when the nurse picks up Violet from her cot and hands her to me. My first reaction is, 'Don't give it to me. What am I going to do with it?' I don't vocalise this thought and instead I just put her to my breast for another excruciating attempt to breastfeed. Soon after I am taking a shower and this is when the tears start. I cry because my scar hurts, I cry because my body has swelled with fluid and I am even bigger than when I was pregnant, I cry because I feel inadequate and overwhelmed, and I cry just because. Chris is a champion. He tells me that it's normal to feel this way and I just need to ride it out.

We go to a community-run information session called 'The First Eight Weeks' a couple of days later. At the session, we have to introduce ourselves to the other parents and talk about our birth stories. I don't know why, but as I talk about my C-section my eyes well with tears. On a rational and intellectual level I don't care that Violet came into the world via the emergency exit. But I feel emotionally wounded by it. All my life I've been told I have childbearing hips and all my life I've worn vertical stripes and A-line dresses, trying to disguise them. Now was their moment to shine and they failed me. What's the point of having childbearing hips if they can't bear children? Or perhaps the C-section was yet another womanly thing that I wasn't able to do like you're supposed to. I couldn't conceive naturally, I couldn't give birth naturally and, I quickly discover, I can't breastfeed naturally either.

# 28

# BOOBS, BOTTLES AND THE BABY BLUES

I have never felt like such a failure in my life. Due to the blood loss from the C-section and a large dose of antibiotics I was given, I struggle to produce any breast milk, which means I spend eight hours a day for the first six weeks connected to a breast pump. Milking yourself like a cow is as degrading as it sounds. To add to the fun, I also get a yeast infection in my nipples, which lasts for two months. The pain of labour is nothing compared to having thrush in your nipples for eight weeks. Labour is excruciating, but it ends. The pain of breastfeeding is the pain that just keeps on giving. And then the mastitis starts, an infection from a blocked milk duct. The first time, I am so ill I am admitted to hospital. After that, I carry antibiotics around in my handbag so I can treat it as soon as it starts. But, of course, the side effect from the antibiotics is another dose of nipple thrush.

Conceptually, I love the idea of breastfeeding. Could there be anything more intimate? But my experience is the exact opposite. I look at my watch and feel sick because it will be time to breastfeed again soon. Then I feel guilty because it's supposed to be a bonding experience. I should just give up and spare myself the pain and anguish. But I know that the sense of guilt and failure at giving up will hurt more than the pain of breastfeeding. I am so guilt-ridden at the thought of giving up that even people's support and compliments weigh upon me like heavy burdens. When my mother says she's proud of me for persisting with breastfeeding despite all my problems, I interpret that to mean that she will be ashamed of me if I stop.

I thought the social pressure to breastfeed wouldn't affect me, but I don't have the strength to stand up against all the breastfeeding propaganda and the mother-bashing that goes on when people can't or won't breastfeed. For a couple of weeks my nipples are so damaged that I can't breastfeed, so I express milk on the hideous milking machine and give it to Violet in a bottle. Even then I can't make enough milk, so I have to supplement most feeds with some formula. Every time I give her a bottle out in public, I feel like I'm being stared at and judged. I'm sure I am overreacting, most of the time, but on one occasion I swear I overhear one middle-aged woman say to another, 'That baby's a little young for a bottle, don't you think?'

Hearing about the experiences of other mothers doesn't help. 'I will never understand women's selfish reasons behind their decision not to breastfeed, even though I understand it is their decision to make,' writes one mother in a parenting magazine. With 'understanding' like that, who needs people to judge you? Calling a mother selfish is surely one of the very worst insults you could ever lay on her. Motherhood is hard enough without people like this kicking you when you're down. Establishing breastfeeding is one of the toughest things I've ever done in my life. And the only reason I can do it is because I have a team of people supporting me. For the first few weeks, Chris takes care of everything while I sit on a breast pump day and night. If you don't have a partner, or your partner is at work all the time, or you have other children to look after, or a job, or whatever, how can you possibly do this? I also attend breastfeeding school twice, pay for a private lactation consultant and spend a fortune consulting a range of doctors – including 'the world's leading expert on nipple thrush'. Imagine having that printed on your business card.

My friend Michelle didn't even attempt breastfeeding. For her, it was a mental-health issue. She'd been through IVF and felt so violated by the experience that she just needed her body back. I have so much respect for Michelle's strength of character. She copped social disapproval from all directions – midwives, friends and complete strangers – but she didn't cave in to the pressure. Her justification was 'happy mummy, happy baby'. Surely Michelle should be applauded, not judged and scorned, for knowing what's best for her and having the resolve to go with her instincts rather than trying to appease others. The best advice I am given comes from a midwife with kids of her own and a lifetime of experience. 'Breast is best,' she says, 'but sometimes bottle is even better.' There is a place reserved in heaven – the one I'm not sure I believe in – for that woman.

The baby blues come and go over the next couple of weeks. Without warning and without any apparent trigger, I turn into a blubbering mess. Every time I catch my reflection in the mirror, I cry some more. I am so swollen I don't look like myself any more. I can't even fit into my maternity clothes, so I spend my days wearing pyjamas or Chris's tracksuit.

But once I get the hang of breastfeeding and learn the skills of mothering to a level where I feel that Violet will neither starve nor die due to my incompetence, I start to love motherhood. I feel completely fulfilled by it and don't want to do or be anything other than a full-time mother. It's one of those rare moments of contentment when you can look at your life and say that there isn't anything else in the world you'd rather be doing than what you are doing. This state of pure bliss lasts for about two months.

When Violet is about five months old, a sense of discontent sprouts within me, and over the following weeks it takes root. I miss my old life. I feel lonely, isolated, bored and boring. I have become one of those excruciatingly dull parents who has nothing to say about anything other than my child. When I catch up with friends, I struggle to contribute to the conversation, partly because I'm so tired that I have trouble concentrating, but mostly because I don't have anything else in my life other than Violet. The only things I can speak about with any authority are Violet's sleep habits and when I'm planning to start introducing solids. Pre-motherhood, when I socialised with friends we spent a lot of time talking about our jobs. But nobody wants to hear about my job any more because my job is mothering. Ours is a society that only cares about mothering when it's selling cleaning products or blaming mothers for either overindulging or neglecting their children, sometimes both at the same time.

Oh, the guilt! I can barely admit my growing sense of discontentment to myself, let alone face the shame of admitting it to anyone else. So I don't. I let it fester for weeks, until one day Chris asks me what's wrong and it all comes out. 'I'm a bad mother,' I sob. 'I'm such a failure as a mother and as a woman,' I sob some more. 'I'm so lucky to have Violet and she's absolutely divine. How dare I want anything more in life?'

Chris looks at me as if I'm crazy and says, 'Of course you want more. Why wouldn't you want all the things you had before?' I know this makes perfect sense. Before I had Violet, I had needs for social interaction, recognition and achievement and personal space. It is bizarre to think that these desires would evaporate or be superseded by the needs being met by motherhood. I know that it's normal to grieve for the things I have lost. How could I not know this? I've read all the literature on it. I just hoped that somehow it wouldn't apply to me, that somehow I'd be different. It seems I have made the same mistake as so many of the women I'd read about when I was researching motherhood; I have confused loving my baby with loving motherhood.

There is no doubt that I feel lay-down-your-life love for Violet, but the process of motherhood is a different story. Just as my friend Sophie wrote in her email all those months ago, sometimes motherhood is pure delight and wonder, but so much of the time it is monotonous, backbreaking, lonely and thankless work. Even as I type this, I have alarm bells ringing in my head: 'What happens when Violet grows up and reads this book and discovers that caring for her didn't totally fulfil me? Will she misinterpret it to mean that I didn't love her enough or that I loved her less than children who have mothers who are completely fulfilled by motherhood?'

My sense of guilt and worry is allayed slightly during an appointment with a psychologist. She says, 'Do you want Violet to grow up with the same unrealistic expectations of motherhood that you had?' She points out that Violet will look to me to learn how to be a woman. What I do is so much more powerful and influential than what I say. 'Do you want Violet to grow up believing that a woman has to sacrifice her own needs for everybody else? That she doesn't deserve to have her needs met or to be a fully rounded and happy human being?' the psychologist asks.

'Of course not,' I say.

'Well then, maybe her mother needs to stop believing it first.'

Chris and I sit down and work out what we can do to help me reclaim a little bit of my life. Of course, I can't have the freedom and autonomy I had before. I don't expect that. But since Violet's birth, I haven't had any autonomy. I have had no pre-planned, non-negotiable time for myself. I have a stolen hour or ten minutes here and there when Violet is sleeping or Chris isn't working. But any plans I make have only been in pencil because if Chris has to do some work or Violet is needy then I cancel them. What I miss the most is the acknowledgement that my time and my plans are important too. Chris leaves the house at the same time each day to go to work, without question. It doesn't matter what sort of night we had or whatever else is going on. He goes to work because his work is important. But my work at the moment is writing. Isn't my work, and therefore my work time, important too? I'm not sure when I'll go back to the corporate world. I was made redundant when I was pregnant, so I don't actually have a job to go back to. I was devastated by my redundancy at the time, even though I had a baby on the way, or perhaps it was *because* I had a baby on the way. I was visibly pregnant and knew that I wouldn't be able to get another permanent job before the baby arrived. I also knew that if I hadn't been doing IVF I wouldn't have lost my job. I would have been able to do the job that required weekly travel and therefore been fully engaged when the axe of the global financial crisis fell. My redundancy was an entrée into the career sacrifices that motherhood requires. But even if I had a job to go back to, I'm told that even mothers in structured work environments experience a devaluation of their work and their time compared with their partners. It's the mother who usually has to take time off when the kid is sick and can't go to childcare. It's the mother who can't work late at night or at the weekend because of the kids. I suppose this is why there is a mummy track and not a daddy track.

Until such time as I get a job back in the corporate world, Chris and I agree that I will have set writing times each week. We mark it in our diaries and agree that, except for exceptional circumstances, I will leave the house and go to work at set times. To make this arrangement work, Chris has to work less. Since Violet's arrival, the number of hours Chris spends working have skyrocketed. Don't get me wrong, he's home early almost every night and all weekend. It's just that when he's at home he has his nose and his attention in his computer. He's present in the house, but I feel like he's often absent from our lives. When I point this out to Chris, he is horrified. He didn't realise I felt this way.

When we talk about it some more, Chris confesses that he feels an incredible pressure to provide. He's been working so hard in order to secure his position at the university until he gets tenure and, eventually, promotion. He worries that he's not earning enough money for our family. But he is. We're making ends meet. But in Chris's mind, he needs to start saving for Violet's university costs and her wedding. Apparently this is quite common for new fathers. They go into provider mode. While this is admirable, I think it's important to recognise that providing for a family is more than just financial. Chris agrees, and I notice that the workaholic has left the apartment and my husband has returned.

# 29

# BAREFOOT IN THE KITCHEN

Although I am leaving the house for a few hours a week to be a writer, when I come home I'm a 1950s housewife. I have become one of those mothers you'd expect to see on the back of a cake packet, except that my husband seems to have been remiss in providing me with a wardrobe full of big flouncy dresses and I still can't bring myself to iron his shirts. Actually, now that I think about it, I can't bring myself to iron anything.

Sometimes I feel like I've changed so much I hardly recognise myself, like when I catch myself barefoot in the kitchen with greasy hair that I didn't have time to wash, let alone dry, slicked back into a ponytail, wearing a tracksuit that is splattered in a cocktail of baby food and vomit, and baking something for dinner. And there are plenty of times since those early days and weeks when I sob in despair at my feelings of inadequacy and loneliness, and grieve for the loss of control over my time, my body and my mind.

Even now, after a year of motherhood, I'm still struck by the yawning chasm that has opened between who I always thought I would be and who I have become. Some days I fantasise about returning to the corporate world just so I can go on a business trip and have a night off. In the evening, I could walk into a hotel room that isn't littered with toys and there would be no basket of dirty washing I'd feel compelled to launder.

191

The work of motherhood is relentless, thankless and, most of the time, invisible. And it is often mothers who downplay and devalue their own status. I am shocked to discover that the worst offenders in stripping mothers of their status and value are not men, and not even childless women: they are mothers themselves. I despair when I hear my new mother friends say that they feel bad that their husbands have to go to work all day and they get to 'swan around at home' or that they feel worthless and powerless because they aren't 'contributing' to the family. Comments like this are stark reminders of just how far we haven't come.

Despite managing teams of people and multimillion-dollar budgets in my professional career, and thinking that I knew a thing or two about hard work, stress and responsibility, nothing compares to the responsibility of motherhood. I have never worked so hard in my life. I have never been so tired and so stretched to my limits. And I am quite certain that my performance has never been judged and critiqued so harshly and by so many people. My friend Sophie says that the hardest part of motherhood is the lack of recognition. But how can we expect our work and achievements to be recognised by other people when we don't even recognise them ourselves?

When I am out in cafes or the library writing this book, people often ask me who is looking after my baby. When I tell them that she is with Chris, they almost invariably reply, 'You're lucky.' And I do feel lucky. But why should I? Should I feel lucky that Chris is taking responsibility for looking after his own child? Are our expectations so low that any time our partners care for their children should be seen as a gift to us for which we should feel grateful? Has Chris ever been asked when he's sitting in a cafe writing who's looking after Violet? And if he had, do you think people would tell him he's lucky that his baby is being looked after by her mother? Not likely. A friend who has recently had her second baby tells me how hard it is to care for two children. Then she adds, 'But I'm lucky, because my husband will look after the girls so I can take a shower.'

Occasionally when I've challenged my friends on the way they devalue their work and therefore themselves, they've replied, 'Yes, but my husband hates his job and I really enjoy being a mother.' But whether you like your work or not doesn't change the fact that it's still work, it's still hard and it is still deserving of recognition and status. In the early days of my career, I loved being a management consultant. But I didn't for a moment think that what I did was less important and less valuable than the work of somebody who hated their job. The two things are not related. But in the world of mothers, we blur the distinction even further with the fact that we feel lucky to be mothers and are grateful to have children.

Compounding this, we also devalue one another through competition. We can't help but look at other mothers and compare their mothering skills and values with our own. There is an unspoken competition over who is the better mother – who is more skilled and who is willing to make the bigger sacrifice for the sake of their child. One mother asks me how much Violet weighs. I tell her I can't remember. And I really can't. I haven't slept for months; I can barely remember my address. Then she asks if I am too embarrassed to tell her because Violet is so chubby. Another mother tells me that she is glad she never gave in and gave her child a dummy. At the time, Violet is sitting on my lap sucking on her dummy. And yet another mother tells me that she would never feed her child commercial baby food. She makes her son's food fresh and only with organic produce. A couple of days later, I bump into her in the supermarket. She is in the baby-food aisle with a trolley littered with commercial baby food.

I'd like to say that I'm different, but I'm not. I'm ashamed to say that I'm just as bitchy and judgemental as everyone else. In the supermarket, I see a toddler throwing a massive tantrum. The poor mother looks completely ragged, she has bags under her eyes so large it's like she has the complete set of luggage under there and she looks like she's about to burst into tears. She grabs a bag of lollies from the shelf and gives it to her kid to shut him up. Before I can help it, I've judged her. I think about all the theories of discipline, and rewarding a tantrum with lollies is not recommended in any of them. I am such a cow. How dare I judge this poor mother? I have no idea what her situation is. It's as bad as people judging me for giving Violet a bottle when they have no idea how hard it is for me to breastfeed.

I can't speak for other women, but the speed with which I judge other mothers comes from insecurity. I desperately want to be a good mother, and the concept of 'good' only makes sense when there is 'bad'. When I see another mother doing something that I wouldn't choose to do, instead of respecting her decision, or feeling sympathy because she's having a hard time, I'll secretly and guiltily feel better about myself. My own insecurity is soothed by the knowledge that I may be a bad mother, but at least I'm not as bad as her. I'm surprised and disappointed by how insecure motherhood has made me.

One of the worst manifestations of competitive mothering is the Smug Mother: the mother who tells anyone who'll listen that mothering is easy and thinks that any woman who complains is just whingeing or attention-seeking. She's the one who claims that motherhood is 100 per cent total joy, that she's never once felt isolated, overwhelmed or bored, and that all those endless sleep-deprived nights of comforting a screaming baby is nothing but a privilege. She's the one who makes me, and almost every other mother that I know, question our mothering abilities and self-worth. If mothering is so easy, why do I sometimes find it so hard?

I'm a big believer in the sisterhood, but I swear, every time I come across a Smug Mother I just want to slap her. Let's go back to Chapter 9 for a moment and remind ourselves that between 50 and 80 per cent of women with young children suffer severe emotional distress on a regular basis. If motherhood is a breeze, then why are women with young children more likely to suffer from depression or be diagnosed with mental illness than during any other time in their lives? I'm not sure if Smug Mothers are just liars and behind closed doors they fall to pieces sometimes too, like the rest of us. Or perhaps they are just really, really lucky to have a baby that has read the manual on feeding and sleeping, and to have family, friends or paid childcare to support them and give them a break so they can stay connected to the rest of the world. If you are this lucky, then please remember that most of us aren't. And if you don't mind, a little empathy wouldn't go astray.

All throughout the emotional roller-coaster ride I've been on for the past year, I'm pleased to say that after the first few days when I felt disconnected from everyone, including myself, I am overwhelmed by love, joy and wonder every time I look at Violet. When the anti-epidural midwife who seems to specialise in drug-free sheep births asks how my birth went and I tell her I had an epidural and a C-section, she says, 'I'm sorry to hear that.' She probably fears that I have failed to bond with my lamb and might accidentally leave her in a paddock somewhere when I go off to munch on some grass. But she need not worry. Violet is the most perfect creature I've ever seen, and I can't believe that we almost didn't – and then almost couldn't – make her. I still have to pinch myself when I think that Chris and I made a person. I feel enriched by motherhood in ways that are beyond expectation and beyond words. One emotion that I can name, however, is relief: I am relieved that I love Violet and I love being her mother.

Let's face it: motherhood is a risk. You have no way of knowing if you're going to like it until it's too late. It's the egg of life that can't be unscrambled. There are times when I long for my old life. A life where I could leave the house without preparation and planning, where I could sleep in and have my own time to do whatever I want and whenever I want, where I am free from the constant worry about Violet's well-being and my responsibilities as a mother. I know this is vain, and I wish I didn't, but I miss my old body. I hate that my boobs are saggy like poached eggs, that I will forever be scarred from my C-section and stretch marks, and that my tummy has a squishiness that won't seem to go away. On the eve of Violet's first birthday, I'm still wearing my maternity jeans. The curtain lady was right: tactless, but right. The weight doesn't come off with breastfeeding. Well, in fairness, all but the last 8 kg fell off without me even noticing. But a surplus of

8 kg is a big enough barrier to prevent me from fitting into my pre-pregnancy clothes and also from feeling good about my appearance.

But during the hard times – and there have been plenty – when I am deprived of sleep, adult conversation and the freedom to just walk away, I am comforted and bolstered by the knowledge that this is the life I chose. I gave motherhood a lot of thought and I went into it with my eyes wide open. I knew about the inequality and the physical, emotional, financial, professional and relational costs of motherhood, and I still chose it freely. I chose it because, out of all the options I had in my life, I wanted to be a mother more than anything else. Hopefully this will sustain me through the tough times and make me cherish the wonderful times even more. Of course, a child is for life and I can't be sure how I will feel in one, ten or twenty years' time. But as I am approaching the first anniversary of my new life, I can tell you that, without a doubt, marrying Chris and having Violet were the best two decisions I've ever made.

# EPILOGUE

I got my happy ending, but what about everyone else?

Emma married Matt in an intimate beach wedding. It was a perfect day: perfect weather and perfect atmosphere. Emma looked beautiful beyond words and Matt looked hot in his open-necked shirt and bare feet. Their wedding vows to each other would have made even the most cold-hearted, unromantic grump shed a tear.

Emma tells me that she and Matt will start 'working on it' when they return from their honeymoon. I'm still not convinced that there is a lot of cluck in Emma's fuck; however, she says that the idea of motherhood is 'growing on her' and she's getting increasingly excited about the prospect. She's seen me do a complete 180-degree turn in the last couple of years and is expecting she will do the same. 'When I see the love that Violet brings to your family,' Emma says, 'why wouldn't I want that?'

When I ask her what she's going to do if she discovers she doesn't like motherhood, she replies, 'I'm hoping biology will kick in. Most people don't hate their children. But if I do, I'll get a job that involves a lot of travel and Matt can raise them.'

It's been almost two years since we met the gorgeous Sharon and Murray at the IVF counselling session and they still haven't been able to have a baby. After each unsuccessful IVF cycle, Sharon says she will give up because she can't go through the stress of yet more injections, drugs and dashed hopes. But, inevitably, she changes her mind and goes back for another roll of the fertility dice. Murray has remained optimistic throughout. He's sure it will happen eventually. Sharon is not so sure. If she's not pregnant within a year, she's going to look into egg donation. She's hoping her sister will donate one of her eggs.

IVF has taken its toll. 'It's difficult catching up with people, because every time I do they tell me they're having a baby or say something insensitive or inappropriate,' Sharon says. Recently a friend was crying on Sharon's shoulder because she'd had unprotected sex for two months and she wasn't pregnant yet. After Sharon consoled her, the friend said, 'When it happens for me, how would you like me to tell you?' So now Sharon just doesn't see anyone. I don't see much of her any more either. After she lost her baby and my pregnancy was progressing well, she told me that it was too painful to see me. I understood completely, so I kept my distance. I bumped into her in a cafe soon after Violet was born. Violet was sleeping in my arms and Sharon could barely look at her. We said a hurried and awkward hello and goodbye and she rushed out of the cafe. I just know that she would have burst into tears as soon as she was out of sight. There's no justice in fertility. Why should I be so lucky to get a baby on my first IVF cycle when Sharon and so many other women try for years without success?

Sharon's story is one more reason we shouldn't buy into the Hollywood fantasy of conceiving effortlessly in our late 30s or 40s, or believe our well-meaning friends when they tell us that we've got plenty of time. Sharon met Murray when she was 35. Soon after they met, Dr Lucy gave her the same 'now or never' speech she'd given me. Dr Lucy told her that she didn't have any time to waste and she should start that week. 'But we'd just met,' Sharon said. 'If I'd gone home and said that to Murray, he would have run a mile and I would have been back to square one.' At age thirty-seven, Sharon started fertility drugs and at thirty-seven and nine months, she started her first IVF cycle. 'And here I am. I'm 39 and childless, and it's flown by,' she said.

Sharon is not the only one who hasn't had her Hollywood ending.

My friend Mary from the meditation dinner party was unable to have a baby and knows now that she'll never be able to have one. At the time of the dinner party, Mary was about to start her first IVF cycle. She did two cycles. After the second cycle, she felt exhausted. She could barely walk to the end of the street and constantly had a feeling of tightness and anxiety in her chest. She would drive door-to-door to work because she didn't have the energy to walk and then come home and lie on the couch all evening. She assumed that it was grief, because by this stage she was 42 and it was dawning on her that her window of opportunity to have a baby had closed.

'Of course, when I read in the papers about the wonder-children conceived by post-menopausal women, I would cling to the hope that it could still happen for me,' she tells me over coffee. 'But deep down, I knew that I wouldn't be able to have kids. I knew the statistics. I knew how unlikely it was to conceive at my age.' Her health deteriorated for five months to the point where she felt ready to die. But aside from the grief, eventually Mary was diagnosed with deep vein thrombosis and a pulmonary embolism. There is some speculation that it was caused by the hormones used for the IVF. Mary's troubles didn't end there. Next, a cyst was discovered on her ovary and the doctors were concerned that she could have ovarian cancer. This led to a hysterectomy and a definite end to Mary's hopes of becoming a mother.

Mary says that she is largely over her grief, but she is still in recovery, both physically and emotionally. 'I've accepted it now, but I still have my moments. I don't think the baby switch has gone off, but I am starting to think about doing other things with my life. At least I did it; at least I tried. It helps to be able to say, at least I had a go.' She's just bought a gorgeous puppy. 'My surrogate child,' Mary says. 'It's such a cliché, isn't it?' The puppy will help her fill her big house. 'The house is too big for me,' she said. 'It was the family home that never happened.'

Linda, the CEO who was pregnant at the time of the meditation dinner party, now has a lovely little boy named Isaac. Linda found it difficult to go through IVF on her own. 'Not only did I not have any support,' she said, 'I also had to hide it. On my fourth IVF cycle, miscarried at work. I felt it happening, but I was in a meeting, so just had to continue on and told nobody. Then I went home to ar empty house. My father had died a month before. It was a pretty low weekend. But during the low times, I just had to remind myself why I was doing it.'

Linda's corporate status brought other challenges that most of u don't have to deal with. When a CEO gets pregnant, it's everyone' business. A CEO is responsible for maintaining the culture and th confidence in an organisation, so knowing that she would be out o action when the baby was born was an 'issue' that needed to b 'managed'. She didn't realise beforehand just how much her pregnancy announcement would affect the entire organisation. She told th chairman, who then called an emergency board meeting. The boar devised a strategic communication plan, the kind you might expec when there is a sudden and massive drop in profits or when mas redundancies are about to be announced. First, the board briefed a the managers in the organisation. Then all the managers mad announcements to all of their staff at the same time. 'I was in m office, knowing that at that particular time the entire organisation wa being told about my pregnancy,' Linda says.

It just goes to show that even when you're at the top of the tree ir an organisation, you can't outrun gender. Can you imagine ar emergency board meeting being called when a male CEO announces he's going to become a father? Rather than worrying about company morale or the confidence of stakeholders or shareholders, peopl instead concern themselves with the type of champagne they shoule send. Women will never be treated equally in the workplace until mer evolve wombs and are capable of bearing children.

Linda's experience makes me realise that even if you are able to buck the trend and have a high-powered career and be a mother, you still have to sacrifice some career satisfaction. Linda is a CEO for billion-dollar company. If any mother would be immune, you'd think he would be. But even she says that she struggles with knowing what he's capable of at work and knowing that she's unable to do it.

'I know I could do more, but I don't get the time and I don't have the energy to do it,' she tells me as we catch up one Saturday afternoon t her beautiful house. 'I've become less creative at work and more me-poor.'

Despite her experiences, Linda is trying to have another baby. She ays she's doing it for Isaac. Because he's an IVF baby and he doesn't ave relatives on his father's side, there is a big chance that he'll end p on his own. 'It was such a big adaption from single career woman o single mum,' Linda says. 'I don't think having another baby will be hat big of an adaption.

'But you need a lot of strength to do this on your own,' she says. 'm a strong person, I'm financially secure, and through Vipassana 'm also more emotionally secure. My life is not tougher than that of single mother on the breadline. With my job, I have the money to fford help.'

I asked her if she would do things differently if she had her time ver. She tells me she would have done it sooner. 'I regret that I left it oo late to find a partner,' she said. 'I should have got over my break-p earlier.'

Kerry, the management consultant who was pregnant at the neditation dinner party, also had a little boy. She named him Ronan. Kerry talks gratefully about the support of her family. 'No one really aises a child alone. Ronan is very well loved by his uncles, aunts and ousins.' Kerry shared a house with her brother for the first nine nonths of Ronan's life, but now she and Ronan live alone. Her mother s chief babysitter and cares for Ronan on Mondays while Kerry vorks. 'Mum's the first one I tell about Ronan's development,' she ays. 'Like the first time he pooed in a potty.'

Kerry is already completely open with her son about his father and lways plans to be. She's connected with the parents of his half-siblings other children conceived with the same donor sperm) via a donor ibling registry. The families share sibling photos, health information

and developmental milestones. 'It's like an extended family. I'd lov
Ronan to develop friendships with his half-siblings in time, if h
wants.' Some of the families are meeting up in Disneyland later in th
year. Kerry is also open with people who need to know, like doctors
and people who are important in her son's life. Surprisingly, Kerry ha
never been asked who the father is. If it comes up, she has a prepare
answer. She'll simply say, 'I'm single and a mother by choice.'

Before Ronan, Kerry thought that having a baby on her own wa
unbelievably brave. She no longer sees it this way. 'It's the best decisio
I've ever made. Motherhood did take a while to get used to. It was
slower pace, more mundane. But I'm enjoying my little guy eve
more than I expected. I did it at the right time, at 36. I'm glad I didn
wait until I was 40.' She is currently pregnant with her second chil
also conceived through IVF with the same sperm donor.

Fleur the sculptor is currently undergoing training to be a respit
foster carer. She feels like she's had a good life and now it's time to giv
something back. She also wants children in her life. 'I love childre
and being around them,' she says. 'It brings out my creativity an
childlike characteristics, and it will also stop me from getting too se
in my ways.' Fleur is going into fostering with her eyes wide open. Sh
expects it to be challenging, particularly when she has to give th
children back. However, it will be an opportunity for her to practis
the Vipassana principle of impermanence and learning how to avoi
feelings of attachment.

Lynn, the marketing executive, is single and still does not have an
intention of being a single mother by choice. Yet she says she admire
the men and women who have the courage to raise their own childrer
'And, while I am choosing not to have children of my own, I believ
I'm doing my part to leave all children a better world.'

Motherhood should be more about choice and less about chance
When you consider that the average life expectancy is approximatel
80 years, we have a relatively tiny window in which to conceiv
children. By pure chance, Dr Lucy brought this to my attention befor
it was too late. I'm one of the lucky ones. Whether you want childre

r not, I believe we should all take the time to gaze out of that window
while it's still open. We spend so much of our lives taking control and
planning for almost everything except children. And tragically, for
many of us, by the time we pull our heads out of the sand of our
careers, our house renovations and our overseas holidays, the window
s closing or has already shut.

# SUGGESTIONS FOR FURTHER READING

Badinter, Elizabeth, *The Myth of Motherhood: An Historical View of the Maternal Instinct* (Souvenir Press, 1981)

Barrett, Nina, *I Wish Someone Had Told Me: Realistic Guide to Early Motherhood* (Academy Chicago Publishers, 1997)

Boulton, Mary, *On Being a Mother: A Study of Women with Pre-school Children* (Tavistock Publications, 1983)

Buttrose, Ita & Adams, Penny, *Motherguilt: Australian Women Reveal Their True Feelings About Motherhood* (Penguin Group, 2005)

Cain, Madelyn, *The Childless Revolution: What It Means To Be Childless Today* (Perseus Books, 2002)

Cockrell, Stacie, O'Neill, Cathy & Stone, Julia, *Babyproofing Your Marriage: How to Laugh More and Argue Less as Your Family Grows* (Collins, 2007)

Craig, Lyn, 'Children and the revolution: a time-diary analysis of the impact of motherhood on daily workload', *Journal of Sociology*, Vol. 42, No. 2 (June 2006)

Defago, Nicki, *Childfree and Loving It!* (VISION Paperbacks, 2005)

Dell, Diana L. & Erem, Suzan, *Do I Want to Be a Mom?: A Woman's Guide to the Decision of a Lifetime* (McGraw-Hill Professional, 2003)

Evenson, Ranae J. & Simon, Robin W., 'Clarifying the relationship between parenthood and depression', *Journal of Health and Social Behaviour*, Vol. 46 (December 2005)

Friedan, Betty, *The Feminine Mystique* (Del Pub Co., 1963; reprint 1984)

Gager, Constance T. & Yabiku, Scott T., 'Who has the time? The relationship between household labour time and sexual frequency', *Journal of Family Issues* (2009)

Gottman, John, *The Seven Principles for Making Marriage Work* (Orion, 2000)

Hakim, Catherine, *Key Issues in Women's Work: Female Diversity and the Polarisation of Women's Employment* (Routledge-Cavendish, 2004)

Hays, Sharon, *The Cultural Contradictions of Motherhood* (Yale University Press, 1988)

Houghton, Diane & Houghton, Peter, *Coping with Childlessness* (Unwin Health, 1987)

James, Oliver, *Affluenza* (Vermilion, 2007)

Kitzinger, Sheila, *Ourselves as Mothers: Universal Experience of Motherhood* (Doubleday, 1992)

Kitzinger, Sheila & Price, Jayne, *Motherhood: What it Does to Your Mind* (Rivers Oram Press/Pandora List, 1988)

Manhaimer, E. et al., 'Effects of acupuncture on rates of pregnancy and live birth among women undergoing in vitro fertilisation', *British Medical Journal* (2008)

Marsh, Nigel, *Fat, Forty and Fired* (Piatkus Books, 2006)

Mattes, Jane, *Single Mothers by Choice: A Guidebook for Single Women Who Are Considering or Have Chosen Motherhood* (Times Books, 2002)

Maushart, Susan, *The Mask of Motherhood: How Becoming a Mother Changes Everything and Why We Pretend it Doesn't* (Random House, 2006)

Morrissette, Mikki, *Choosing Single Motherhood: The Thinking Woman's Guide* (Be-Mondo Publishing, 2005)

Nicolson, Paula, *Postnatal Depression: Facing the Paradox of Loss, Happiness and Motherhood* (John Wiley & Sons, 2001)

Pape Cowan, Carolyn & Cowan, Philip A., *When Partners Become Parents. The Big Life Change for Couples* (Basic Books, 1992)

Simring, Steven, Klayans Simring, Sue & Busnar, Gene, *Making Marriage Work for Dummies* (John Wiley & Sons, 1999)

Tanenbaum, Leora, *Catfight: Rivalries Among Women – From Diets to Dating, From the Boardroom to the Delivery Room* (Harper Paperbacks, 2003)

Vargo, Julie & Regan, Maureen, *A Few Good Eggs: Two Chicks Dish on Overcoming the Insanity of Infertility* (ReganBooks, 2006)

Walsh, Denis, 'Pain and epidural use in normal childbirth', *Evidence-based Midwifery*, Vol. 7, Iss. 3 (September 2009)

Winnicott, Donald, *The Child, the Family and the Outside World* (Penguin, 2000)

# ACKNOWLEDGEMENTS

This book may never have been written if Brandy Walton hadn't sent me an email suggesting the title and commanding me to start writing it. Thank you to Brandy for the constant encouragement and for reading every single draft. And this book would not have been published without the enthusiasm and hard work of the talented people at Mainstream Publishing. Many thanks. Thank you also to my agents, Jane Graham Maw and Jennifer Christie, for their ongoing support and hard work.

The inner world of motherhood, infertility and assisted reproduction spins on an axis of secrecy, guilt and shame. Thank you to all those people who were brave enough to tell me the whole truth and allowed me to 'out' them in the pages of this book. I haven't listed you by name because some of you are more 'out' than others. Please know that I am honoured and grateful for your honesty, humility and humour.

Thank you to my trusted advisors and friends for their encouragement, constructive feedback and babysitting offers, and for allowing me to use them as sounding boards: Elodie Andrieu, Sarea Coates, Sarah Coghlan, Jules Cole, Deb Cox, Kate Edwards, Stephen Farquhar, Katie Foat, Tessa Kitchener, Cindy Lau, Emma Lindsay, Rebecca Lowth, Melissa McLean, Nadia Michaelides, Sonya Michele, Gabriela Fiorese Neilson, Alyson O'Shannessy, Jen Rae, Jamie Rossato, Willow Sainsbury, Cheryl Taube, Tracy-Jean, Rachael Tricavico-

Smith, Alanna Vaz and Stephanie Zemanski. Thank you also to my family for their support and proofreading: Michael Edwards, Wesley Edwards, Jan Edwards, Valerie Scanlon and Frank Scanlon. I am indebted to all the people who read my previous book, *30-Something and Over It*, for their support and encouragement. Thank you for giving me the confidence to do it again.

Since I don't have a room of my own in which to write, I turned the front table at Eurodore cafe into my office. Thank you to Nicole Rabbito for always remembering my coffee order and to Peter Moutis for not charging me rent.

Thank you a hundred times over to Christopher Scanlon. Most men would not even share with their doctors the information that I have revealed about him in this book. I could not ask for a more loving, fun and supportive partner in my life, or a more ruthlessly constructive editor and brilliantly funny joke doctor in my work.

Of course, the last words are for my darling Violet. What a gift you are. I never knew I could feel so much.

\*       \*       \*

Kasey Edwards is a change management consultant and the author of *30-Something and Over It: What Happens When You Wake Up and Don't Want to Go to Work . . . Ever Again.*

She has recently acquired a husband and a daughter. Her poodle is unimpressed.